Tell Me What to Eat if I Have Type II Diabetes

by

Elaine Magee, M.P.H., R.D.

ROSEN PUBLISHING

New York

This edition published in 2009 by:

The Rosen Publishing Group, Inc.
29 E. 21st Street
New York, NY 10010

Design by Nelson Sá

Library of Congress Cataloging-in-Publication Data

Magee, Elaine.
Tell me what to eat if I have type II diabetes / By Elaine Magee.
    p. cm.
First published as Tell Me What to Eat if I Have Diabetes by New Page Books/Career Press.
Includes index.
ISBN-13: 978-1-4042-1835-2 (library binding)
1. Non-insulin-dependent diabetes—Diet therapy. I. Title.
RC662.18.M34 2009
616.4'62—dc22

                                         2008015245

Table of Contents

Introduction 7

Chapter 1:
The Who, What, Where, Why,
and How of Type II Diabetes 9

Chapter 2:
Top 7 Profiles of Type II Diabetics 19

Chapter 3:
Everything You Ever Wanted
to Ask Your Dietitian 43

Chapter 4:
The 10 Food Steps to Freedom 75

Chapter 5:
The 26 Recipes You Can't Live Without 117

Chapter 6:
Navigating the Supermarket 157

Chapter 7:
Restaurant Rules to Eat By 181

Chapter 8:
Smart Snacking 201

Conclusion 213

Glossary 215

For More Information 217

For Further Reading 219

Index 220

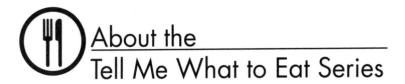

About the
Tell Me What to Eat Series

The Tell Me What to Eat series is not about telling you which foods you can't have. It won't lecture you, or tell you to spend hours preparing all your foods from scratch. Above all, no matter what the ailment, the Tell Me What to Eat books give you nutrition you can live with—literally. It is food and nutrition that will help you live longer and feel better and it is also practical and enjoyable enough that you actually want to live longer.

These books are about you and how you like to live and eat. One of the first things each book does is answer your most pressing questions about what to eat. People like to take supplements—you will find advice about supplements. People like to eat at restaurants and in fast food chains—you will find realistic advice about this too.

Most people who suddenly find themselves dealing with a disease or syndrome just want to know the minimum of information to get by—to feel better. In my work I often hear people say, "Just tell me what to eat." What they are really saying is, "Don't tell me about all the different studies, the theory, and scientific hypothesis surrounding it. I don't need to know why as much as I need to know what and how to eat."

Whether you're researching headaches and migraines, type II diabetes, or how to help prevent breast cancer, the Tell Me What to Eat series will always stand for practical, realistic, understandable diet advice—nutrition you can live with.

Ⓘ Introduction

I t would have been much easier to write this book if there was one specific diet to recommend for all persons with type II diabetes. But there isn't. The truth is all persons with type II diabetes are not created equal. Each person needs to work out his or her particular eating, exercise, or medication plan that translates into normal blood sugars in their particular body. Some people seem to have better blood sugars with meals low in fat while others do better with meals richer in monounsaturated fat (30 to 40 percent calories from fat). But no matter which type of person you are, you will still need the tools to be able to count the fat and carbohydrates into your meal plan. We'll give you those tools. There are other food patterns and nutrients that seem to help most people with diabetes. We'll talk about that too.

Most diabetes specialists believe there are three keys to managing diabetes:

1. Monitoring your blood glucose levels.
2. Exercising regularly.
3. Following your personalized eating plan.

This book, *Tell Me What to Eat If I Have Type II Diabetes,* will obviously spend the bulk of its pages on the third key. But don't be surprised if you find some tips on the first two as well. As a matter of fact, exercising regularly and monitoring your blood glucose are two of the 10 Food Steps to Freedom in Chapter 4.

In the past, it was mainly overweight adults who developed type II diabetes. However, doctors are now finding that more kids and teens are developing type II diabetes. This is probably the case because more kids and teens are overweight.

I hope, as you read this book, you will feel as though I am holding your hand and walking with you as you begin this journey. I know how difficult and sometimes depressing having type II diabetes can be. I have held my dad's hand through the last 20 years of having this disease. He wasn't interested in helping his body live longer and better with this disease. But hopefully you are. I wrote this book to help you.

The best gift I can give you is to approach life as if you don't have diabetes—for many this includes eating foods you love and enjoy. This book will get you closer to that goal. That is my promise.

Chapter 1

The Who, What, Where, Why, and How of Type II Diabetes

Diabetes is reaching epidemic proportions. It is the third or seventh leading cause of death in the United States, depending on whether you include the people with diabetes who die from related cardiovascular disease. Roughly 18 million Americans already have diabetes and many more will get it in the coming years as baby boomers age and the rise in adult and child obesity continues. Experts say that about eight to nine million Americans are walking around not knowing they even have diabetes. Often they don't find out until fairly severe damage has been done to their bodies. What kind of damage? Diabetes is the leading cause of blindness, kidney failure, and leg amputations.

Once you have diabetes, your risk for heart disease can be four times greater. So telling you what to eat for type II diabetes also has to include telling you what to eat to reduce your risk of heart disease. In fact, the types of food and meal choices that work best for diabetics (lower sugar, lower sodium, high fiber, fruits, and vegetables, with sources of monounsaturated fats and omega-3 fatty acids) is great for someone without diabetes. The only difference is that people with diabetes need to carefully control and monitor their blood sugar and therefore sometimes need to keep count of carbohydrate, fiber, and fat grams throughout their day.

The bottom line then for most people with type II diabetes is eating good food at good times in good portions. That's what the rest of this book is all about.

Who is at risk for type II diabetes?

- People age 45 and older.
- People with a family history of diabetes.
- People who are overweight.
- People who do not exercise regularly.
- Certain racial and ethnic groups (African Americans, Hispanic-Americans, Asian-Americans, Pacific Islanders, and American Indians).
- Women who have had gestational diabetes or who have had a baby weighing 9 pounds (4.1 kilograms) or more at birth.

What exactly does insulin normally do in the body when the body isn't resistant?

Insulin is a hormone normally produced as needed by the pancreas, and one of its major jobs is helping get glucose (energy) into various body cells. When blood glucose levels rise, the pancreas makes more insulin and releases it into the bloodstream. The insulin then causes body cells to remove the excess glucose that is circulating in the blood. In the liver and skeletal muscle cells, the insulin encourages the production of glycogen (the storage form of glucose). In the liver and fat cells, insulin encourages fat production (stored energy). At the same time insulin discourages the breakdown of body fat for energy (lipolysis), causing the body to rely more heavily on the recently ingested carbohydrates for current energy needs.

What is type II diabetes?

Type II diabetes is a metabolic disorder resulting from the body's inability to make or properly use insulin. (Insulin is a hormone that converts sugar, starches and other foods into energy.) It occurs when the body produces plenty of insulin, but the insulin cannot do its job. For some reason, the cells in the body have become resistant to insulin. In most cases, being overweight or obese for a period of time could bring on the insulin resistance. But there are people who are obese for many years who never develop diabetes. So scientists suspect that some people have a genetic predisposition (their particular family genes make them more likely to develop type II diabetes under certain conditions such as with aging, weight gain, or an inactive lifestyle).

Ninety to 95 percent of people with diabetes have type II. About 5 to 10 percent have type I (usually diagnosed among children or in young adults, and usually not associated with obesity).

What are the warning signs of type II?

Often people with type II don't have obvious signs. But they could also have any of the following traditional type I symptoms:

- Frequent infections.
- Blurred vision.
- Cuts and bruises that are slow to heal.
- Tingling/numbness in hands or feet.
- Unusual thirst.
- Frequent urination.
- Extreme hunger.
- Unusual weight loss.
- Extreme fatigue.
- Irritability.

Why do people get type II diabetes?

Not all persons with type II diabetes are created equal. It acts differently in every person. But most people with type II diabetes start with the potential to develop the disease (genetic predisposition), based on family history or ethnicity, that eventually becomes manifest through environmental factors such as aging, weight gain, or a sedentary lifestyle.

What are the end-points of diabetes?
Diabetes is the leading cause of blindness in working-age adults in the United States, accounting for 24,000 new blind persons every year. The National Eye Institute estimates that 90 percent of lost vision is preventable.

- Diabetes is the leading cause of end-stage renal disease in the United States. Approximately 28,000 patients with diabetes develop end-stage renal disease every year. With all the current therapies now available, future cases of end-stage renal disease are probably preventable.

- Diabetes is the leading cause of nontraumatic lower extremity amputations in the United States.

How will this book help?
I know it takes some time to really accept that you now have diabetes. This may take a few months or a few years, depending on the person. A good friend of mine was in what you could call "diabetic denial" for about two years—not exercising, not really paying attention to her blood glucose or what she ate. I wrote another book called *The Good News Eating Plan for Type II Diabetes*, and she was one of the first people to whom I gave a copy. Every time I would see her, I would ask if she had read it. She would always have an excuse.

Finally one day she said, "I guess I better start acting like a diabetic." Almost overnight she started monitoring her blood glucose, counting carbohydrates, fat and fiber, and working some exercise into her busy workweek. She feels much better now. Guess what? She had finally read the book.

If you are reading this book right now, chances are you are there. You have accepted that this is now a part of your life. You want to make it work for you. You want to manage your blood glucose, reduce your risk of heart disease, and just plain feel better. Then and only then can this book help.

 How can I manage my diabetes?
Many diabetes specialists believe there are three keys to diabetes management success:

1. Monitoring blood glucose levels.

You need to monitor your blood glucose because that's how you know right away if you are keeping your blood glucose near normal. And you need to keep you blood glucose near normal if you want to protect your body from developing diabetic complications further down the line. If your healthcare team knows how your blood sugar is being affected from day to day, they can help fine-tune your medications, your eating plan, and your exercise routine.

Measuring your blood glucose will tell you rather quickly whether your treatments (diet, exercise, and pharmacological) are working for you. Make sure someone on your healthcare team clearly demonstrates how to measure your glucose and how to record it so it can be referred to easily at follow-up visits.

This is very important to the management of diabetes. Next to the discovery of insulin, the ability to monitor blood sugars was the biggest breakthrough in the treatment of diabetes.

2. Exercising regularly.

Exercise can actually help control blood glucose levels. Exercise depresses insulin production and also prompts skeletal muscle cells to take in more glucose from the blood-stream. With more glucose in your muscle cells, you can produce more energy so that your muscles can continue to work).

Besides helping to control blood glucose levels, exercise improves the cardiovascular system (thus reducing the risk of heart disease) and also encourages weight loss, which can have big benefits for people with diabetes.

3. Following a personalized eating plan.
Follow a plan that helps keep your blood glucose levels normal, helps protect against heart disease and weight gain, and doesn't make you feel deprived. This is the key that this book will give you the most help with.

This book, though, is not about telling you the one and only way to eat—no one diet is best for all people with diabetes. Every person has different risk factors (obesity, hypertension, high triglycerides, kidney dialysis, etc.) that need to be considered. I will tell you generally which foods or meals will be more likely to cause higher blood sugars. But when it comes right down to it, every person is affected by the same food or meal a little differently. Chalk it up to unexplained individual differences.

F.Y.I.   Losing Weight

Weight loss in people with type II diabetes results in the following health benefits:
- Reduced endogenous production of glucose.
- Increased peripheral insulin-mediated glucose uptake.
- Increased release of insulin.
- Improved insulin sensitivity.

NOTE: Weight loss greater than 5 percent also improves cardiovascular risk factors, dyslipidemia, and high blood pressure.

(Diabetes, Obesity & Metab. 4:415-423. 2002)

Generally, many people with diabetes seem to tolerate a more moderate carbohydrate (around 45 percent calories from carbohydrate), moderate fat (around 35 percent calories from fat) way of eating. Of course this eating plan requires using mostly canola and olive oils and avocado (which are high in more desirable monounsaturated fats), and having a couple servings of fish (rich in omega-3 fatty acids) a week wouldn't hurt either.

An Aspirin a Day ?

Atherosclerosis, vascular thrombosis, and platelet abnormalities all contribute to cardiovascular disease in people with type II diabetes. (People with type II diabetes produce more thromboxane, and aspirin blocks thromboxane synthesis.) Several large-scale trials have shown aspirin to be of significant benefit for primary and secondary prevention of cardiovascular events in diabetic patients. One of the trials using male physicians showed that the group of diabetics reduced the number of heart attacks (myocardial infarctions) from 10.1 percent (placebo group) down to 4.0 percent with 325 mg of aspirin taken every other day.

Given the possible benefits of aspirin therapy, the American Diabetes Association Clinical Practice Recommendations (ADA, 2000) suggest using enteric-coated asprin (81 to 325 mg per day) for secondary prevention in diabetic patients with large vessel disease and for primary prevention in diabetic people at increased risk (positive family history, tobacco use, obesity, dyslipidemia, hypertension, albuminuria, and age greater than 30 years).

Recommendations for Aspirin Therapy:

Lipids:
- Cholesterol greater than 200 mg/dl.
- LDL cholesterol greater than or equal to 100 mg/dl.
- HDL cholesterol less than 45 mg/dl (men), less than 55 mg/dl (women).

- Triglycerides greater than 200 mg/dl.
- Age older than 30 years.

Use enteric-coated aspirin in doses of 81-325 mg/day. (Diabetes Care 26 [suppl 1]: s87-s88. 2003)

Before you add aspirin to your day, talk it over with your doctor. There are some people who shouldn't consider aspirin therapy: those with aspirin allergies, bleeding tendencies, recent gastrointestinal bleeds, liver diasease, active ocular bleeding, and people on anticoagulant therapy or taking ACE inhibitors with established cardiovascular disease, and people younger than 21 years of age shouldn't take aspirin on a regular basis due to an increased risk of Reye's syndrome.

Where can I go for more information?

- To find a certified diabetes educator in your area (many provide individual consultations and some offer classes for diabetics), contact the American Association of Certified Diabetes Educators toll-free at 800-832-6874.
- For a list of registered dietitians with expertise in diabetes (RD, CDE) in your area, contact the American Dietetic Association's National Center for Nutrition and Dietetics at 800-366-1655 or visit it's Website www.eatright.org and click on "Find a Dietitian."
- The American Diabetes Association maintains a hotline at 800-DIABETES (800-342-2383) and information on types of diabetes is available by mail, fax, and staff members. The association's Website is www.diabetes.org.

Hopefully your local diabetes center or clinic has a referral sheet available, filled with local numbers for everything from diabetes support groups and counselors to dietitians, diabetes educators, fitness clubs, and personal trainers. If they don't, find someone who does. Many hospitals have diabetes support groups, and that is a great starting place.

This chapter was reviewed by:
Joseph Barrera, MD, Medical Director
Alta Bates Diabetes Program in Berkeley, California

Chapter 2

Top 7 Profiles of Type II Diabetics

I know you feel like you have been wearing this label "type II diabetes" lately and that health professionals and other people like to lump all type II's together. The truth is that people with type II diabetes come in different shapes and sizes and with different health risks and medical problems. Your health risks and medical problems, in addition to having type II diabetes, also define what needs to be done food-wise to help you feel better and live longer. It is important we get these other issues on the table so that you can get a better idea of what your personal diet and food priorities are and how your type II diabetes might differ from others.

There are certain trends that stand out in people with type II diabetes. I've attempted to talk about many of these trends in this chapter. Maybe you will find yourself described in one or more of the following profiles.

1. Waiting to lose weight

Let me first say, you are not alone. I have spent most of my adult life waiting to lose weight. I understand how difficult it is. I know that often thin people actually eat more and exercise less than thicker people (but who's counting?). I know what it is like to eat healthy, exercise every day, and still not lose weight. I have even been told I am too fat to talk about eating healthful on television. But I am the most common size in America—I am a size 14.

One third of Americans are considered "overweight." But what shocked me was that survey data (National Center for Health Statistics) in 1988-1991 showed a dramatic increase of about 8 pounds in mean body weight of U.S. adults since the previous survey was conducted (1976-1980). It didn't matter which gender, age, or cultural group you looked at— weight gain still followed.

How can this be? Jenny Craig, Weight Watchers, Slim Fast, and other billion dollar dieting giants have been waging war against weight gain for decades now! Never before have more reduced-fat foods been available. Getting back to the basics of weight control sheds some light on this rather sore subject.

As you've probably heard, one of the first questions related to weight control is do the "calories in" equal the "calories out"? That's because the net effect of excess calories (more than our current body needs), even in the form of carbohydrates or protein, is going to increase the amount of fat put into storage (body fat). We know that most Americans haven't exactly been increasing their "calories out" side of the equation. Due to a combination of modern life factors (television, long commutes, computers, etc.), Americans have become more sedentary.

What about the "calories in" portion? True, the average person ate less fat as a percentage of total calories during the survey period (from 36 to 34 percent)—but the amount of total daily calories went up an average of 231 calories compared to 1976-1980. Aaah . . . now we're getting to the real million-dollar question. Why would Americans suddenly increase their total daily calories at a time when the country has never been more obsessed with dieting and more concerned about healthy eating?

Ironically, some researchers think it is exactly this over-emphasis on fat-free foods that has contributed to the rampant weight gain. Perhaps this wave has fed the belief that if a food has little or no fat, you can have as much as you want without gaining weight. Perhaps when people eat mediocre fat-free foods, it leaves them feeling unsatisfied, so they eat more of the fat-free products, or end up eating something else in hopes of satisfying their hunger or food craving. Maybe because a large chunk of the American population is actively dieting at any one time, they continue to ride the unfortunate weight roller coaster of strict dieting and obsession—deprivation, bingeing and guilt, strict dieting and obsession—over and over again. Studies show that when people diet the vast majority of them eventually gain the weight back—and then some. Maybe some of these 8 pounds are the "and then some" from a country that chronically diets.

So what are we going to do about it?

- *Stop Dieting!* We know it doesn't work. We know it actually works against you.

- *Eat when you are hungry and stop when you are comfortable.* When we "diet" we force ourselves not to listen to our natural hunger cues. When we do this, we also tend not to listen to our "comfortable" cues. We react to deprivation and not listening to hunger by overeating at times. In order to stop overeating, we need to stop dieting and start listening to when our body truly is hungry and truly is comfortable.

- *Start Exercising!* Exercising helps your body in so many ways. It is one of the fastest ways to increase your "calories out" side of the equation. (See Step #10 in Chapter 4 for information about how to exercise if you don't like to exercise.)

- *Start Counting* carbohydrates, fats, and fiber as often as you can to gain close control of your blood sugars. I know counting is a big pain. But you don't have to do it all the time for the rest of your life. You might start counting your carbs, fat, and fiber every day until your blood sugars are under control. Then you can do "check in" counting— about every week or every month if your blood sugars are staying within normal limits.

Logging in what you eat and your exercise will also help you and your dietitian or certified diabetes educator better understand what small changes might take place to encourage weight loss. Granted, all of the above are easier said than done.

To diet or not to diet

When the holidays have finally passed, 'tis the season to get dieting. It's the American way. But when it comes to shopping for a "diet," it's buyer beware, according to a new report from the Federal Trade Commission, released September 17, 2002. The researchers found that 55 percent of the weight-loss advertisements made at least one false or unsubstantiated claim. Does this really surprise us? Nearly half the ads claimed you could lose weight without dieting and exercise.

All fad diets promoting fast and furious weight loss generally don't work over the long haul. Some of us have already figured this out on our own but we can't quite stop ourselves from perking up and asking "How'd you do it?" every time we hear someone say they lost 20 pounds. We can't quite tune out the countless TV commercials we see daily for weight-loss programs and products.

If you are going to partake of a fad diet in the new year, go in forewarned that with fad diets, weight loss is temporary. A USDA study found that pretty much any fad diet will help you take off the pounds, but there's not much evidence that they'll help you keep the weight off. Fad diets often work in the short run because they are low calorie diets in disguise.

Weight loss fact: The only way to lose weight is to consume less energy (calories) than your body needs. No magic ingredients or food combinations will change this basic metabolic fact.

But most people who successfully lose weight return to their old eating habits sooner or later and regain most of the lost weight within two years (Am J Cardiol 2001;88:59-61, Denke M. Metabolic effects of high-protein, low-carb diets). That's why (nobody wants to hear this) the diet or way of eating you choose needs to be practical and healthful for a lifetime. Most fad diets are not.

The fact is (nobody wants to hear this either) there is no miracle remedy or diet for losing weight. Your best bet is to stick with the proven method of eating less, eating healthier, and exercising more.

So say you are ready to try to eat less, eat healthy, and exercise more. Which "diet" or way of eating is the best way to do that? The popular low carb/high protein way? The low-fat/higher carb way? Or, the moderate fat way (but emphasizing the better fat, carb, and protein choices). Each will work in the short run as long as the calories you take in are less than the calories you are expending. But healthwise which is best?

Health Test #1: Where are the fruits and vegetables?

Instead of "Where's the beef?" one crucial question to ask when looking at these different diets is, "Where are the fruits and vegetables?" Recent studies have shown that the obesity levels are lowest among those who eat seven or more servings of fruits and vegetables a day (key finding from new research from the Produce for Better Health Foundation, Press Release October 21, 2002). And perhaps it isn't a coincidence that as Americans have been getting fatter over the last 10 years, fruit and vegetable consumption has declined nearly 14 percent, nationwide, during the same period. We all know fruits and vegetables are good for us, well guess what...they are mostly carbohydrate (vegetables will have some plant protein too).

A cup of steamed broccoli contains 44 calories, 4.5 grams protein, 8 grams carbohydrate, .5 grams of fat, and 4.7 grams of fiber. And a large apple contains 125 calories, .4 grams protein, 32 grams carbohydrate, .7 grams of fat, and 4.2 grams fiber. Both are brimming with a good dose of healthful carbohydrate, complete with fiber.

Health test #2: Are you losing fat, lean body mass, or body water?

No one will argue that the main goal of weight loss is to lose body fat weight and not lean body mass (muscle). Water loss is fast and temporary, so eventually your body is going to need to restore the balance of water and will gain lost water pounds back.

When you are eating a low carbohydrate/restricted protein diet, some body protein is broken down to provide glucose energy so valuable muscle mass will actually decline on this type of diet. The ideal weight loss diet should provide enough carbohydrate to prevent this protein/muscle breakdown, enough good quality protein to meet the normal needs of protein turnover, and enough fat to meet essentail fatty acid requirements.

The following covers each of these three major "diet" groups, their strengths and their weaknesses, and some tips for you to keep in mind, should you decide (after consulting your doctor or dietitian) that's the program for you.

High protein/low carbohydrate. This type of diet does encourage fast weight loss in the first week. Though what's initially happening here is mostly water loss. The body needs a constant supply of glucose energy, so without a lot of carbohydrates in the diet, body glycogen stores (the way the body stores some extra carbohydrates) are used up. For each gram of glycogen lost, 2 to 4 grams of body water is lost as well. One study demonstrated that the greater weight loss on a low carbohydrate/high protein diet plan is accounted for by losses in body water (Am J Cardiol 2001;88:59-61, Denke M. Metabolic effects of high protein, low carbohydrate diets).

The American Heart Association has officially cautioned the public on high protein diets. In an advisory to clinicians, it concluded that people who follow high-protein diets are at risk for "compromised vitamin and mineral intake, as well as potential cardiac, renal, bone, and liver abnormalities overall" (Circulation, 2001, Vol. 104, No. 15, pp. 1869-74). According to this American Heart Association Science Advisory report, "the beneficial effects on blood lipids and insulin resistance are due to the weight loss, not the change in caloric composition." The advisory also reminds us that there are no long-term scientific studies to support the overall efficacy and safety of the various and sundry high protein diets (including Atkins, the Zone, Protein Power, Sugar Busters, and Stillman).

The one plus with this type of diet is that you can lose weight fast, which can give some people the impetus they need to make more longer term changes in their eating habits and lifestyle. But losing weight too fast can be a problem too. When weight loss is too fast, changes in body composition, especially the loss of lean body mass, can compound the problem of overweight in the long run. When you lose weight fast, you tend to lose some lean body mass (muscle protein), but when you gain the weight back fast, it tends to come back as mostly body fat.

The other plus: There is some evidence that higher-protein diets are more satiating. People feel fuller and tend to eat less after a meal with a high protein content (over 25 percent calories from protein). High protein foods tend to move more slowly from the stomach to the intestine than high-carbohydrate (refined) foods, so your stomach tends to feel full longer.

Of the five high protein diets on the market, two score slightly better nutritionally than the others. The Zone and Sugar Busters diets at least do not severely restrict carbohydrate to less than 100 grams a day and total fat and saturated fat are not excessive (greater than 30 percent calories from fat and 10 percent calories from saturated fat). (Circulation, 2001, Vol. 104, No. 15, pp 1869-74.)

The bottom line: This way of eating can't and shouldn't be continued over a long period of time. These diets are generally associated with higher intakes of fat, saturated fat, and cholesterol, because the protein is provided mostly from animal sources. In the long term, very high protein diets may increase the risk of atherosclerosis (one study showed that this diet increases serum cholesterol levels and may increase the risk of coronary heart disease by more than 50 percent with long term use (J Am Coll Nutr 2000; 19:578-590). Dr. Thomas Lee, M.D., commented in the March 2002 issue of the Harvard Heart Letter that for most people eating a high-protein diet (including lots of cheese, red meat, and other high fat foods), their cholesterol levels, especially LDL (bad) cholesterol, go way up and that limiting foods that lower LDLs (such as high fiber plant foods) only intensifies this problem.

Here's another fact that you need to keep in mind with high protein diets: The more protein you eat, the more calcium you excrete. High protein diets, when followed for a long time, can increase your risk of osteoporosis by increasing calcium excretion, and place an extra stress on the kidneys (which are removing high amounts of nitrogen waste products from the high protein intake, particularly during times of high water loss from perspiration or low fluid intake contributing to dehydration.)

Short term consequences of following a diet that encourages high protein and fatty foods include dehydration, diarrhea, weakness, headaches, dizziness, and bad breath. This type of diet also tends not to include sufficient fruits and vegetables for overall good health.

High carbohydrate/very low fat: The biggest positive to this type of diet is that it can lead to healthy eating as long as the diet recommends high fiber intakes, lower glycemic index carbohydrates (fruits, vegetables, beans, and whole grains tend to have lower glycemic indexes), and provides sufficient essential fatty acids and fat-soluble vitamins from the fats that are eaten.

Another plus is that the diet quality tends to be better with this type of diet compared to the low carb diets. A recent U.S. study of popular diets demonstrated that the diet quality (measured by dietary variety and intake of five food groups, fat, saturated fat, and sodium) is higher in high carb diets and lowest in low carb diets. The same study also detected another plus to high carb eating: The body mass index (BMI) is lower in people following high carb diets and highest in people on low carb diets (JADA 2001; 101:411-420, Kennedy et al., "Popular diets: correlation to health, nutrition, and obesity").

The trouble with a high-carb/low-fat diet is that some might be tempted to fill up on higher glycemic index carbs (refined starchy foods and concentrated sugar), which are rapidly digested and can cause a large increase in blood glucose and insulin after meals. Some clincial trials have reported less weight loss on high glycemic index diets compared to low glycemic index diets and some short-term feeding studies found that as glycemic index goes down, satiety (a satisfied feeling of fullness) tends to go up. (Obes Rev 2002 Nov;3(4):235-43, Pawlak et al., "Should Obese patients be counselled to follow a low-glycemic index diet?")

The bottom line: Choose mostly smart carbohydrates (higher fiber, higher nutrient carbohydrates with lower glycemic indexes) and make sure you are getting enough protein and fat (olive oil, canola oil, fish, etc . . .) to meet your body's needs.

The moderate, balanced diet: This more moderate, balanced way of eating tends not to be studied as a "diet" so there is very little research on this type of diet and weight loss. But if you combined the best part of the high-carb diet with the best part of the high-protein diet would you have the best of both worlds? In one study, a low-fat diet with 25 percent calories from protein was found to produce a significant reduced calorie intake and greater weight and fat loss over a six-month period compared to a low-fat diet with a lower protein intake—12 percent calories from protein (Int J Obes Relat Metab Disord 1999; 23:528-536). That sounds encouraging.

If this way of eating emphasizes the higher fiber, nutrient-rich carbohydrate foods (whole grains, beans, fruits, and vegetables) and the lower-fat protein sources (lean meats, fish, skinless poultry, low-fat dairy, and/or vegetable protein sources such as beans, whole grains, nuts and seeds) and uses some of the more favorable cooking fats (olive oil and canola oil), this diet is clearly the best of both "diet" worlds.

What to look for in a weight-loss diet

- Does it consider your current habits, preferences, and risk factors?
- Does it set realistic weight loss goals (1-2 pounds per week)?
- Does it have a daily intake of at least 1,200 calories for women and 1,500 calories for men?
- Does it have a carbohydrate intake of at least 150 grams per day?
- Does it include all of the food groups?
- Does it emphasize fiber?
- Does it recommend regular exercise?
- Is it based on changing life-long eating habits?

The bottom line

Do your "calories in" equal your "calories out"? No matter which diet you are on, the bottom line is always that the net effect of excess calories (more than our current body need), even in the form of carbohydrates or protein, is going to increase the amount of fat put into storage (body fat). Most Americans haven't exactly been increasing their "calories out" side of the equation. Which leaves us with the "calories in" portion. Recent surveys have shown that we have reduced our percentage of calories from fat a tiny bit, but they have also shown that we are eating more calories per day!

2. I have couch potato-itis

If the first thing doctors told you to do (after being diagnosed with type II diabetes) was "lose weight," then the second thing they probably told you was to "start exercising." The bottom line is that physical activity can make the difference between losing weight and not losing weight, blood sugar control and out-of-control blood sugars, going on insulin and not having to go on insulin, taking a high dose of insulin and taking a lower dose of insulin. Regular exercise has been shown to lower high triglycerides levels in the blood and lower high blood pressure after only 10 weeks. The risk of heart attack also decreases with regular exercise.

Exercise does much more than reduce risk factors; it has psychological benefits, too. It just plain makes you feel better. It tends to encourage better sleep, and it gives you more energy throughout the day. It helps you feel better about your body even if pounds haven't been lost, and it helps reduce depression and stress.

I can go over and over all the various and sundry benefits (immediately and down the road) of exercise and physical activity, and I can even hold your hand and follow you around for a month helping you get in the habit of exercising. But sooner or later it is all going to come back to one person—you. There is only so much others can do. Ultimately you have to take responsibility for yourself.

The first step, other than accepting that you have diabetes, is to commit to trying "exercise" for 1 month, remembering to start slowly. To see major benefits in your blood sugar control, exercising five to six times a week (even if it is just for 15 minutes each time) is helpful. At the end of one month you should hopefully have experienced many of the psychological and physiological benefits to exercise and you will be, let's hope, adequately "hooked." So let's look at how to get started:

- Visit your doctor and make sure you can proceed with your plans to start exercising.
- Don't make it a big weight loss contest—focus on health and gaining better control of your blood sugar.
- It has to be fun or you are definitely not going to stick with it.
- Find out what your exercise preferences/needs are and try to consider them when making your exercise plans.
- Do you like exercising outdoors or indoors?
- Do you like to exercise alone, with a partner, or with a group?
- Do you like the gym atmosphere?
- What time of day would you be most likely to stick to exercising?
- Do you have any physical limitations that need to be considered? If you have joint limitations, for example, water aerobics or swimming can actually be a great starting place.
- What do you like to do? Even if your answer is watching television or talking, they can be worked into your exercise program. If you like to talk, walking with a partner might be the ticket. If you like to watch television, then home exercise equipment that you can do in the comfort of your family room or bedroom might be your most practical option.

Every little bit helps

Even if you can't imagine exercising 30 minutes or more in one sitting, split it up into 3 10-minute mini-workouts. Ten minutes of activity here and there does add up to health benefits for your body. Any way that you can increase your activity throughout your day will help your cause.

Tips to keep you exercising month after month

- Wherever you choose to exercise (gym, park, or pool) it should be no more than 20 minutes away from your home or work.

- Start an exercise journal or incorporate the information into your food freedom journal. You will be able to see progress. You will also be able to trace back situations when the exercise helped lower your blood sugars.

- Have a plan B. Have some indoor options for exercise planned. During the winter, it might be too cold to exercise outdoors, or it might get dark earlier and you are concerned about safety. Or perhaps you get stuck in traffic and don't get home in time to make your exercise class. Your plan B could be riding your stationary bike or playing one of your exercise videos.

- Plan variety into your exercise schedule. If you go to a dance class two times a week, you might want to add a walking workout a couple times a week. I have three different types of exercise I do in any week (what can I say, I get bored easily). I go to jazzercise two to three times a week and fill the rest of my week in with walks around the neighborhood and evening rides on my stationary bike (while I watch my favorite nighttime television shows.)

- Make different types of activity part of your normal day. These may include walking the dog, walking to the mailbox, taking a flight of stairs, or walking during part of your lunchbreak.

- You can "check in" with a personal trainer every three months. They can give you specific things you can do, given your personal experiences and preferences. A "check in" session will run you about $30 to $100 and you can call the American College of Sports Medicine for a list of personal trainers in your area.

- To keep yourself from getting bored, don't be afraid to try something new. You could sign up for a class with your local parks and recreation program or through a community college. You could try a session of country western dance class and then try yoga, water aerobics, tai chi, or tap the next session.

- You've got to choose exercise that you actually enjoy. Of course it is a matter of personal preference, but a large majority of people enjoy walking the most. It's easy, free, and only requires a pair of comfortable shoes. Look around your home or work for lakes or parks that you can walk around after dinner, during the lunch hour, or on the weekends.

Home Exercise Equipment

Stationary and recumbent (when your back is supported) bicycles are very successful with former couch potatoes. You can literally go from the couch to the bicycle. Position a fan in front of the bicycle if you like. There are a few things to consider when picking out an exercise bike:

- Make sure the seat is adjusted to your body correctly.

- Make sure the seat is wide and comfortable.

- If you opt for a stationary bike, consider the type where the fly wheel gives you a breeze (helping you to cool off) and the handles move (because this prevents leaning).

- Many people make the mistake of buying the inexpensive exercise equipment. I know this is tempting. To get the well-made equipment, the kind that will last a lifetime, it will run you around $800 (give or take a couple hundred.) This is shocking, I know. But if you buy the cheaper stuff that creaks when you use it, it will inevitably break or you will tire of it quickly because it isn't as comfortable to use. Isn't buying one of the well-made pieces of equipment better than buying three cheaper pieces that you will stop using after a few months? Many stores offer payment plans where the cost is something like $20 or $30 a month.

There are also places that sell used exercise equipment, which would shave quite a bit off the price.

Another home exercise no-no: Don't buy exercise equipment through catalogs or television commercials. You want to try it out before you buy it. Literally get your sweats on and go to the exercise store. Tell them you want to try it out for 20 or 30 minutes. Only then will you be able to tell whether you can comfortably exercise on it for at least 30 minutes at home.

If you want to research the better designed pieces of exercise equipment, look up *Consumer Reports* at your local library—they rate exercise equipment every year. But remember the only way to know for sure how you like it is to just get on and try it.

Exercise videos

I picture exercise videos sitting week after week on a shelf somewhere. But then again, I'm not an exercise video person. I can buy them alright; I just don't ever wind up in front of my television and do it. I'd rather be walking outside or watching a movie or television show while riding my bike. Obviously, some people actually use their exercise videos. In fact, they might even find them motivating. Probably one of the most motivating for larger sized exercisers are the Richard Simmons tapes, which use larger-sized exercisers in the video itself.

You can use videos as a discreet way to try something new (like step classes or kick boxing) in the privacy of your own home. You don't have to worry about what you look like in those jogging shorts or whether you stumble off your "step" in step class because you are the only one there.

If this appeals to you, send for this free catalog, "Complete Guide to Exercise Videos" by Collage (800-433-6769). It lists the tapes by category and tells you exactly what to expect with every video—the type of music, the length, the exercise level, the components of the workout, etc.

There is something for just about everyone—exercise to gospel music, country western dance workouts, and even a hot dance workout video by Paula Abdul.

3. Hyper about hypertension

At least one in every four American adults has it, and about 60 percent of people with type II diabetes have it. Its cause is basically unknown. If left untreated, it can kill you suddenly, without warning. What is this silent killer? It's hypertension (or high blood pressure). If you have hypertension, chances are you are taking some medication to help control your blood pressure, and you might have been told to change your diet in a few different ways. Blood pressure reduction should begin if multiple readings, preferably taken out of the office, are above 130/85 mmHg. Therapy should always include lifestyle modifications, especially weight loss and regular physical activity, even if the doctor has prescribed blood pressure lowering medications.

Tidbits about high blood pressure and type II diabetes

- High blood pressure affects about 20 to 60 percent of patients with diabetes.
- High blood pressure increases the risk of both macrovascular and microvascular complications.
- In one major study, each 10 mmHg reduction in mean blood pressure measurements was associated with:
  - 12-percent reduction in risk for any complications related to diabetes.
  - 15-percent reduction in risk for deaths related to diabetes.
  - 11-percent reduction in risk for myocardial infarction.
  - 13-percent reduction in risk for microvascular complications.
  - Blood pressure greater than or equal to 120/70 mmHg are associated with increased cardiovascular event rates and mortality in diabetics. Target blood pressure goal is less than 130/80 mmHg.
  - Weight loss of 2.2 total pounds has resulted in a mean arterial blood pressure reduction of about 1mmHg.
  - Moderate intensity exercise has been shown to lower blood pressure.

(Diabetes Care 26 [Suppl 1] s80-s82. 2003)

> ## F.Y.I. Who's at risk for hypertension
>
> - The incidence of severely high blood pressure is three times higher for African Americans than for Caucasians.
> - The older you get, the higher your risk. (By age 74, half the U.S. population has hypertension.)
> - If you're considered "obese," your risk is increased.
> - If you're older than 35, use oral contraceptives, and smoke, your risk is increased.
> - If you have diabetes or kidney disease, your risk is high.

If you have hypertension and diabetes, you probably feel like you are taking an entire handful of medications every day to keep your blood sugar and blood pressure in check. But if you are able to improve your blood sugar and blood pressure by eating wisely, you may be able to reduce the dosages for some of those medications (and maybe even eliminate one or two of them.)

Improving your blood pressure, though, isn't going to make you feel "better," like improving your blood sugar does. You will just have to take my word for it. It's a very good thing—a life saving measure. Both of my parents-in-law died, unexpectedly, in their 50s due to uncontrolled high blood pressure. Two of their children are already on high blood pressure medications (one being my husband) and two have borderline high blood pressure and are being closely monitored.

Besides medication, high blood pressure treatment usually includes weight reduction. If you're obese, avoid excess sodium and salt in your diet, and exercise. Guess what? We should be doing most of these things anyway for diabetes and for our general health. There are some minerals, relatively new on the hypertension scene, that may help in the treatment and possibly the prevention of hypertension:

- **Magnesium**: Eat magnesium-packed foods, such as fruits and vegetables, whole grains, and lower fat dairy items, to ensure a good intake of magnesium.

- **Potassium**: A diet rich in potassium (for those without kidney damage or failure) may provide some protection for the arteries of people with high blood pressure. It may also lower blood pressure a little and protect the kidneys from related damage.

    Potassium is the mineral that made the banana famous, but potatoes, apricots, orange and grapefruit juice, and just about any kind of fruit and vegetable not cooked in water (because some of the potassium will pass from the vegetable into the water) will add potassium to our diets. (People with a history of kidney failure should check with their doctors before increasing the intake of potassium-rich foods.)

- **Calcium:** Just when you thought it was best to avoid dairy products, evidence turns up linking decreases in systolic blood pressure (the top number in the blood pressure reading) with higher intakes of calcium or calcium supplements. It seems to work the best in people with previously low intakes of calcium (below the recommended daily allowance) who also have high systolic blood pressure readings.

4. Salt movers and shakers

Here's the deal. About one in five Americans are thought to have a sensitivity to sodium (which is found in many things including salt, MSG, soy sauce, brine, broth, and any compound with the word "sodium" in them such as sodium phosphate.) People who eat out and eat processed foods tend to take in a lot more sodium (and salt). The trick here is that everyone has a different level of salt that they are used to tasting in food. If you are used to quite a bit of salt/sodium in your food, lower sodium items will taste bland to you (temporarily). So restaurants and food manufacturers tend to err in favor of the people used to tasting more salt/sodium in their food. This learned preference for salt takes about two months to unlearn. As you eat less and less salt/sodium, your taste buds become more aware of the salt and sodium that's there—but it takes time so try and be patient.

There's not much you can do about the salt/sodium in restaurant foods and certain processed foods, such as turkey dogs and bacon, and lunchmeats and the occasional frozen entrée. But you can, at least, stop using the salt shaker.

When it comes to salt there are two types of people—the "movers" and the "shakers." The "movers" move the salt shaker to the cabinet and bring it out only if absolutely necessary. Most "shakers" (people who like to shake that salt) usually do so before even tasting the food. If this describes you, then you, my friend, have a bad habit. If you've got to shake something, opt for freshly ground pepper or several of the Mrs. Dash salt-free seasonings. Keep in mind that 1/2 teaspoon of salt is worth 1,000 milligrams of sodium.

5. Type II and thin

There are a small percentage of people who have type II diabetes but they are not overweight. This describes about one in every 10 persons with type II diabetes. Many of these people successfully manage their diabetes with oral medications (not insulin). This makes them similar to other people with type II diabetes, but they don't have many of the other medical problems (extra weight, blood pressure, and elevated blood fats) that are common in the majority of people with type II diabetes.

Thin people with type II diabetes tend to be more sensitive to medications. They may need to pay attention to preventing blood sugars that are too low. It is essential that these people work with a certified diabetes educator or dietitian to fine tune their daily food plan because their greatest challenge may be to find ways to get more calories into their day without throwing their blood sugars off too much.

6. A diabetic on dialysis

Some people with type II diabetes are on dialysis because their kidneys can't do their job anymore. Many of these people experience drastic swings in their blood sugars so they might need to check their blood sugars more often, particularly when they are first getting used to dialysis. You can work with a certified diabetes educator or dietitian when you first begin dialysis to help fine tune how best to eat, based on your dialysis schedule. Your food plan may need to be different on days that you have and don't have dialysis.

If you are on dialysis you need to make sure you are getting enough protein to maintain your lean body mass (which keeps your metabolic rate higher) but not so much that your levels of BUN (blood urea nitrogen) are too high in between dialysis visits. Generally, you are encouraged to eat from .6 to 1.2 grams of protein per kilogram body weight per day (depending on how many times you go to dialysis a week, what type of dialysis, and other factors).

7. Syndrome X—Y me?

Syndrome X, also known as "dysmetabolic syndrome," is basically a collection of certain physical and medical problems. If you have or are at risk of having type II diabetes and you are also overweight, have high blood pressure, and your serum triglyceride levels are too high, you are one of a growing group of people who have what some scientists refer to as syndrome X. Some experts believe the diabetes is only the "tip of the iceberg," with high blood levels (hyperlipidemia), high blood pressure, and coronary disease being the larger part of the overall condition. Believe it or not, it is estimated that 22 percent of the U.S. population has this condition.

I know that, at first, it seems high blood pressure, high triglycerides, obesity, and diabetes are all separate medical problems. But it is quite possible that all of these are actually related to the same metabolic-based problem where there is a disturbance in metabolizing carbohydrates (type II diabetes) and lipids (high serum triglycerides and low levels of the "good" or HDL cholesterol). What causes this metabolic disturbance? We don't really know, but syndrome X is generally associated with obesity. But what comes first, the chicken or the egg—the obesity or the metabolic disturbances?

Diagnosis of dysmetabolic syndrome is confirmed when any three of the following criteria are met:

- Waist to hip ratio is greater than 1.0 in men and greater than .8 in women.
- Serum triglycerides are greater than 150 mg/dL.
- HDL is less than 40 mg/dL in men and less than 50 mg/dL in women.
- Blood pressure is greater than 130/85 mm/Hg.
- Serum glucose is greater than 110 mg/dL.

No matter what the cause, if this describes you, you need to know what type of eating plan tends to work best—higher carbs and lower fat or a more moderate carbohydrate and higher fat eating plan. And the winner is: the more moderate fat diet (rich in monounsaturated fats and omega-3 fatty acids but low in animal fats)—about 30 to 40 percent calories from fat. But will this make you fatter? When the calories going in are kept constant, diets slightly higher or lower in fat do not appear to result in significant weight gain. The trick to eating 30 to 40 percent calories from fat is not exceeding your required amount of energy (calories) and emphasizing monounsaturated fat and omega-3 fatty acids while limiting saturated and trans fats. (See Chapter 3 for more information on higher or lower levels of fat, and check out the A-Z Guide to a Healthy Heart on page 57.)

Chapter 3

Everything You Ever Wanted to Ask Your Dietitian . . .

Diet and Type II Diabetes

Do you have a list of foods I cannot eat?

No—there isn't a list of foods you absolutely cannot eat. All foods, with smaller serving sizes, can be worked into a particular eating plan. If dietitians tell you that you can't have something anymore, it will only make you feel deprived and angry and you will only want to have that food more. You ultimately decide what to eat. And it is you who will learn to associate certain foods in certain amounts and in certain combinations with higher blood sugars in your particular body.

I have a sweet tooth. Can I still eat some of my favorite desserts?

No one wants to be told they can't have something— especially sugar. It only makes you want it more. And there is no reason why people with diabetes can't have sugar, as long as they keep a few things in mind. Bread and several other starches actually have almost the same effect on blood sugar in some people as refined sugar does. The recommendations from the American Diabetes Association basically say if you are managing your blood sugar well, then you may have some sugar—but you've got to play by a few rules:

- *Pay attention to portion sizes of sugary foods.* Keep servings moderate, like 1/2 cup of ice cream or three Oreo cookies.

- *Try to enjoy your dessert or high-sugar treat as part of a meal.* You will be less likely to overeat the treat if you have it with a meal and the dessert will be less likely to send your blood sugar soaring if it's paired with other foods.

- *Substitute the sugar-containing food for another carbohydrate-containing food in your personal diabetes meal plan.* Otherwise you will not only increase the carbohydrates you're taking in, you'll also increase your calories.

- *Monitor your blood glucose routinely so you'll be aware of any negative effects from the sugary food.*

The lesson here: Go ahead and eat cake, but make it a modest slice and have it with your meal. One last bit of advice: Make sure these foods are truly satisfying, so you'll be happy with the moderate amounts.

How can I do this without counting and measuring foods?

I don't like counting and measuring either. It automatically makes you feel "different" (and not in a good way) and frankly it can take the fun out of eating. I would strongly suggest doing some counting of carbohydrate, fat, and fiber grams every now and then just to sort of "check in" with how you are eating. When you compare it to blood sugars, this can be a great tool for you and your dietitian or diabetes educator. But if you really can't bring yourself to do it, the only answer is to monitor, monitor, monitor (your blood sugar that is). Monitor your blood sugar three to six times a day, study your normal diet and the resulting blood sugars, and soon you will know which foods/meals work best.

The foods that do cause high blood sugar may just need to be eaten in smaller amounts each time, combined with other foods, or coordinated with a change in medication or exercise just when that specific food/meal is eaten.

Should I become vegetarian?

A total vegetarian diet can be high in carbohydrates, making normal blood sugars harder to achieve for some. If you choose to eat this way for other reasons, make sure you plan meals carefully to keep carbohydrates in check. You will need to depend heavily on higher protein and fat plant foods such as nuts and soybeans or tofu and plant foods rich in soluble fiber to help buffer the carbohydrate induced rise in blood glucose. What might appeal more to most people is to eat, not necessarily a "vegetarian diet," but to just plain eat more plant foods.

Why is it so important that I eat more plant foods?

"Plant foods" include fruits and vegetables, grains (such as bread, rice, pasta, and cereal), tubers (includes the potato family), and legumes (includes the bean and pea family). As you can tell from the list, these foods tend to be loaded with vitamins, minerals, fiber, and phytochemicals (plant chemicals that have health-promoting properties), most of which help protect against cancer in a variety of ways. Nutrients in plant foods also help protect our bodies from other diseases such as heart disease, stroke, and hypertension. Making plant foods take up a larger portion of our dinner plate can also help reduce obesity.

I've heard there is a type of fiber that is good for people with type II diabetes. What is it?

Soluble fiber (fiber that is soluble or dissolves in water) seems to be a vital component of blood glucose control for many people. It is found in peas and beans, oats and oat bran, barley, and some fruits and vegetables. Soluble fiber leaves the stomach slowly, so it makes you feel satisfied longer. I notice it when I have beans with lunch, such as a bean burrito. (This is unusual becuse I am usually starving several hours after lunch.) Soluble fiber, which forms a gel within the intestinal tract, slows carbohydrate absorption and reduces the rise in blood glucose and insulin following the meal. Soluble fiber also has some disease prevention benefits. Find out more about this is Chapter 4 (The 10 Food Steps to Freedom.)

Q   Are the popular very high protein, very low carbohydrate diets good for people with diabetes?

These diets aren't good for anyone but they can be dangerous in people with type II diabetes. People with diabetes are already at high risk for kidney disease (diabetes increases the rate that the kidneys age) and excessive food protein and high blood pressure put even more stress on the kidneys. These are all just fad diets in disguise—they aren't based on scientific and medical truths. Just think about it: Fruits, vegetables, and whole grains are some of the most nutritious foods on Earth, contributing vitamins, minerals, phytochemicals, and fiber. These foods are made up of mostly what? Carbohydrates. And while it is true that insulin is normally released into the bloodstream when carbohydrates are eaten (in people without diabetes), the carbohydrates are stored as fat only if the amount of calories being eaten is greater than the amount needed by the body. So carbohydrates don't automatically turn to fat unless you are eating too much.

Okay, so people say they have lost weight on these diets. The only thing that really counts is whether they were able to keep it off (and in this respect, people haven't been as lucky.) People may lose weight on these diets not because they are low in carbohydrates, but because they tend to be low in calories. People do lose weight quickly, but it isn't fat they're losing right away; it's mostly body water. As you continue the diet, you will lose some fat pounds, but at the same time, you are losing muscle tissue.

When you eat too few carbohydrates, your body automatically starts to sacrifice its protein tissue (from major organs and muscles) for energy. And when you gain the weight back it is likely as body fat, not muscle tissue. Over time, losing weight and gaining it back a few times causes you to get fatter and fatter and lose more and more muscle tissue. The liver and kidneys also have to work harder processing protein into energy than carbohydrate.

 Are starchy foods such as pasta, potatoes, and bread fattening?

All of these foods are high in carbohydrate calories. Carbohydrates are only fattening when we eat more calories than our body needs. But this is also the case with foods high in protein and fat (especially fat). By including fruits and vegetables with these starches, we are more likely to keep our portions of these delicious starches reasonable. For example, when you fix pasta, add in some broccoli or carrots. When you make a sandwich with bread, have it with an apple, a wedge of melon, or a small bowl of fruit salad. With bread, you also have the opportunity to increase your daily fiber total by choosing bread that either contains whole grains or contains added soluble fiber.

I'm confused. Is fat in food good or bad? I know it's bad with some diseases but I also know it helps me control my blood sugars?

Let me tell you a story. Once upon a time, all that the townspeople knew about food fat was that it tasted good and kept their bodies a little padded so they could better survive the winter and periods when food was scarce. People often cooked their food in lard or shortening. They uninhibitedly spread butter on their bread, corn, and potatoes. People delighted in drinking extra rich milk. Fatty meats and sausages were considered highly desirable. What bliss!

Over the past 15 years, needless to say, things have become much more complicated. Fat in food is feared; its mere presence has been known to inflict massive guilt on people. But the latest studies are showing us that some fats actually have a protective effect on our bodies in terms of heart disease and some cancers. They are also showing that there may not be one "right" amount of fat for all people—some people may fare better with more or less fat than others. Researchers are probably going to battle this out in the years to come but in the meantime you're trying to get a better handle on your blood sugars, your weight, and your risk of heart disease.

I don't blame you for being confused. Most of us health professionals are trying to figure it all out too. Yes, having a moderate-fat diet (30 to 35 percent calories from fat) seems to add up to better blood sugars for some people with type II diabetes compared to a very low-fat diet (10 to 20 percent calories from fat). The fat helps slow down digestion in general, and "paces" the introduction of glucose (from carbohydrates eaten) into the bloodstream. For a variety of reasons, fat also helps some people feel more satisfied after a meal or snack.

The tricky part is knowing how much is enough for the diabetic benefits but not too much that it increases your risk of other chronic diseases as well as weight gain. I would try to stick to around 30 to 35 percent calories from fat and see what effect it has on your personal blood sugars, weight, and blood lipid levels. This way you could still have about 15 to 20 percent calories from protein, leaving around 45 to 55 percent calories from carbohydrates (hopefully mostly from whole grains, beans, fruits and vegetables).

As part of this moderate-fat eating plan you absolutely must turn to the more heart protective fats to make up most of this "35 percent"—the omega-3 and omega-9 fatty acids and the monounsaturated fats. This means using canola oil and olive oil in cooking, choosing products that contain liquid canola oil or olive oil (non-hydrogenated), including flaxseed, enjoying a handful of nuts every now and then, and eating fish a couple times a week.

If you like eating out, these new rules could cramp your style. Most fast food and restaurants do not use liquid canola and olive oil (except maybe an Italian or Mediterranean restaurant). You will learn more about eating out in Chapter 7.

Q Do blood lipids tend to improve after people with type II diabetes emphasize/switch to mono-unsaturated fats and omega-3 fatty acids?

Yes! Some people who achieve good blood sugar control on low fat/high carb diets unfortunately see their LDL "bad" cholesterol and triglycerides increase. But after adding omega-3 fatty acids and monounsaturated fats to about 30 percent calories from fat (or a little more), many people are able to improve their blood lipids without an increase in HgA1c (a blood test that, in essence, measures the 90-day average of blood sugars).

Q The more I incorporate beans into my diet (which helps my blood sugar) the more gas I get. Is there anything I can do?

The fiber and some hard-to-digest complex carbohydrates in beans and legumes end up in the large intestine. The bacteria in the intestine then work on breaking down these substances, often giving off gas as a byproduct, making you feel bloated. There are a few things you can do to minimize the gaseous effects of beans. Keep your serving of beans to about half a cup to start with and eat beans with a balanced meal (containing protein, fat, and carbohydrates). There are also a couple of over-the-counter products that claim to alleviate bean digestive distress. You can give them a try by calling their 800 numbers and asking for a free sample. Try Beano (800-257-8650). It comes in a chewable tablet or liquid to be taken with beans. Or try BeSure (800-527-5200), which comes in a capsule that you take at mealtime.

What about the advertisements I hear for foods and products that help you burn body fat fast, even while you sleep!

To burn more body fat, your body has to require more calories than it is taking in with food. This means exercise, building muscle, and eating a little less than your body requires. You know what they say—if it sounds too good to be true, it usually is. Anybody can tell you anything to help sell a product. For most quick and fast claims, there is no real science backing them up.

You should also avoid buying weight-loss products using "speed" substances such as ephedra, ma huang, guarana, or high doses of caffeine. These may artificially increase your metabolic rate, but can be absolutely dangerous. These substances do not offer any long-term weight-loss advantages and that's what really matters. Try to avoid the temptation of a quick fix. Trimming off extra pounds takes time. Concentrate on eating healthy and exercising, because they benefit your body in many different ways—trimming of extra weight is just one of them.

What are bad and good cholesterol?

A high level of LDL-cholesterol in the blood increases the risk of fatty deposits forming in the arteries, increasing the risk of heart attack. That's how LDL has gotten its nickname as the "bad" cholesterol. Elevated levels of HDL-cholesterol, on the other hand, seem to have a protective effect against heart disease, which is why it has been coined "good" cholesterol. What about "total" serum (blood) cholesterol levels? Many people think lowering food cholesterol is the most important step toward lowering blood cholesterol. Actually, eating less saturated fat has a stronger effect on lowering blood cholesterol levels. Some studies, though, have found that eating cholesterol increases the risk of heart disease, even if it doesn't increase blood cholesterol levels.

What do all those different fatty acid words mean?

Here are brief definitions of key fat-related ingredient and medical terms:

Cholesterol: A chemical compound manufactured in the body. It is used to build cell membranes and brain and nerve tissues. Cholesterol also helps the body make steroid hormones and bile acids. The liver makes all the cholesterol the body needs.

Dietary cholesterol: Cholesterol found in animal products that are part of the human diet. Egg yolks, liver, meat, some shellfish, and whole-milk dairy products are all sources of dietary cholesterol.

Fatty acid: A molecule composed mostly of carbon and hydrogen atoms. Fatty acids are the building blocks of fat.

Fat: A chemical compound containing one or more fatty acids. Fat is one of the three main constituents of food (the others are protein and carbohydrate). It is also the principal form in which energy is stored in the body.

Hydrogenated and partially hydrogenated fat: A fat that has been chemically altered (made more saturated and therefore more solid) by the addition of "hydrogen" atoms. If a vegetable oil is completely saturated or "hydrogenated" it becomes a saturated fat. When a vegetable oil is partially hydrogenated, some trans fatty acids are formed (see trans fatty acid). Margarine and shortening are examples of partially hydrogenated and hydrogenated fats.

Monounsaturated fat: Fat made of "mono" unsaturated fatty acids (which are missing "one" pair of hydrogen atoms in the middle of the molecule—they have one unsaturated chemical bond). Monounsaturated fats are found mostly in plant and seafoods. Olive oil and canola oils are the two high monounsaturated fat oils. Monounsaturated fats tend to lower levels of LDL-cholesterol ("bad" cholesterol) in the blood.

Polyunsaturated fat: "Poly" unsaturated fats are missing more than one pair of hydrogen atoms—they have more than one unsaturated chemical bonds. Polyunsaturated fats tend to lower levels of both good (HDL) cholesterol and bad (LDL) cholesterol in the blood. Safflower, corn, and soy oil are mostly polyunsaturated fats.

Saturated fat: A fatty acid that has the maximum possible number of hydrogen atoms attached to every carbon atom. It is "saturated" or "full" with hydrogen atoms. Saturated fats tend to raise levels of LDL cholesterol in the blood, and elevated levels of LDL cholesterol are associated with heart disease. Saturated fats are naturally found in animal products such as butter, lard, meat, and whole-milk products.

Trans fatty acids: A polyunsaturated fatty acid in which some of the missing hydrogen atoms have been put back in a chemical process called hydrogenation. Trans fatty acids are byproducts of partial hydrogenation. Trans fats may be as dangerous to our health as saturated fats, raising LDL "bad" cholesterol and total cholesterol levels.

Lipoprotein: A chemical compound made of fat and protein. Lipoproteins that have more fat than protein are called low-density lipoproteins (LDLs). Lipoproteins that have more protein than fat are called high-density lipoproteins (HDLs). Lipoproteins are found mainly in the blood where their main function is to carry cholesterol around.

Foods and blood sugars

 How and why do certain foods raise blood sugars more than others do? I find that pizza, for example, causes higher blood sugars than candy?

The foods we eat contain different amounts and combinations of carbohydrates, protein, and/or fat. Vegetable oils contain all fat and granulated sugar contains all carbohydrate. Other foods contain two or three of these. All of the grams of the digestible carbohydrates we eat convert to glucose, while about half of the protein and 10 percent of the fat grams we eat converts to glucose after digestion.

Carbohydrates, protein, and fat show their peak effect on blood glucose at different times after a meal, too:

- Simple sugars—Peak 15 to 30 minutes after the meal.
- Complex carbohydrates—Peak 1 to 1 1/2 hours after the meal.
- Protein—Peaks 3 to 4 hours after the meal.
- Fat—Peaks 3 hours after the meal.

How a particular food affects your blood glucose has to do in part with the combination of carbohydrate, protein, and fat in the food and the portion size you eat. How quickly the food is absorbed (and how quickly it affects blood glucose levels) also has to do with things such as the physical form of the food, whether the food is cooked, and what blood glucose levels were before the meal. One trick all people with diabetes have up their sleeves is dietary fiber. Dietary fiber, which is not digested by the body, causes other carbohydrates in the meal to be digested and absorbed more slowly.

However, people respond differently to carbohydrates. The same meal eaten by different people might have varying effects on blood glucose levels. And in some people, insulin becomes less effective after they eat high animal fat meals. This can also bring on high blood sugars. The only way to know for sure how your blood sugar responds to a particular meal is to test your blood sugar before and two hours after the meal.

 What are the meals/foods that surprisingly encourage higher blood sugars than expected in some people?

Some health professionals call this, "the pizza effect." So you can guess what is at the top of this list—pizza. Other foods that cause many people problems are:

- Chinese food in general (Chow mein in particular).
- Ramen noodles.
- Bagels eaten plain (even one bagel can cause a problem for some). Start with half a bagel and eat it with some peanut butter or light cream cheese.
- Fried foods (such as fried chicken and french fries).
- Granola cereal (start with 1/4 cup).
- Pasta (try a 1-cup serving of cooked 100-percent durum wheat semolina pasta, and start the meal with a soup or salad).
- High animal protein/fat meals (including those with lots of cheese).

 Are there any foods that, when part of a meal/ snack that usually invites high blood sugars, seem to help prevent the higher blood sugars after the meal?

Adding plant foods that contribute some fat and/or protein to the meal (nuts, soyfoods, olive and canola oil, flaxseed, avocado) seems to help minimize high blood sugars from notorious high carb meals. But if you have a meal high in animal fat that usually brings on high blood sugars (pizza, high fat breakfasts, etc.), loading up on fiber (soluble fiber in particular) about 10 minutes before you start the meal may help. Higher soluble fiber plant foods will also help minimize high blood sugars from high carb meals too. As an appetizer (a little before you eat the entrée) try:

- A green salad with kidney beans and raw vegetables.
- A cup of vegetable or bean soup.
- A small serving of oat bran or oatmeal (before a problematic breakfast).
- Other high soluble fiber vegetables (see Chapter 4 for a list).

- Other high soluble fiber grain foods (see Chapter 4 for a list).
- Psyllium seed foods and supplements (powders without intestinal stimulants are available, psyllium is also added to a couple of breakfast cereals).

How come I seem to have higher blood sugars after high-fat meals instead of high-carbohydrate meals?

Some people seem to have high blood sugars after meals particularly high in animal fats such as bacon and eggs or pizza topped with sausage and pepperoni. Some researchers think that in some people (particularly certain ethnicities) insulin becomes less effective after meals laden in animal fat. If you notice this happens with you, try having smaller portions of the fatty foods and add in some plant foods (fruits, vegetables, and grains, especially those rich in soluble fiber) and see if it makes a difference. Instead of bacon and eggs and hash browns, try one sausage link, one egg, and pancakes or a bowl of oatmeal. Trade in your four slices of "animal lover's pizza" for:

- A couple slices of "vegetable lover's" pizza. Plus . . .
- A green salad with kidney beans and a olive oil vinaigrette or a nice cup of vegetable or bean soup to go with it.

What is the percentage of carbohydrates, fat, and protein that seems to help most people with type II diabetes control blood sugars?

According to certified diabetes educators who I spoke with, about 1/3 of the people with type II diabetes tend to do better with an eating plan including around 35 to 40 percent calories from fat (using mostly monounsaturated fats) while 2/3 tend to fair best with a 25 to 30 percent calories from fat. But there are many other food factors, other than the percent of fat or carbohydrates, that can influence blood sugar control, such as total fiber/soluble fiber, and whether proteins and fats come mostly from vegetable sources.

Q Who tends to do better with higher carbohydrate, lower fat meals?

People whose insulin seems to be less effective after high saturated/animal fat meals (which seems to include Asians, Pacific Islanders, and African Americans) tend to do better on a higher carbohydrate eating plan (especially if they are not exercising regularly). Including foods rich in soluble fiber helps many people tolerate a higher carbohydrate meal. (See Chapter 4 for more on soluble fiber.)

Q What is a good breakfast if your blood sugars tend to be high in the morning?

Many people with type II diabetes have trouble with morning blood sugars, not necessarily because of what they ate for breakfast but because their "wake-up" blood sugars started high. Many people tend to be more resistant to insulin in the morning. Start by fixing yourself a nice balanced breakfast, with carbohydrate, protein, and fat. You can do this by adding nuts to cereal and muffins. Some people don't mind adding soy milk or almond milk to their cereals in the morning. If you are having pancakes, serve up a couple slices of turkey bacon. If you are having a bagel, add a slice of ham and cheese, a tablespoon or two of peanut butter, or 1/8 cup of light cream cheese.

Q My doctor keeps telling me that I am at an increased risk for heart disease due to my diabetes. What can I do diet-wise to reduce this risk?

Basically, once you have type II diabetes, your risk for heart disease can be four times greater. That's why the tips and food commandments throughout this book consider heart disease prevention at the same time they cover diet recommendations for type II diabetes.

Some people really feel like they don't have any control over their increased risk for heart disease. There are all sorts of ways that you can help your body resist the progression of heart disease beyond the obvious (controlling your blood sugars). Just to give you an idea of all the things you can start doing today, the following is an alphabet's worth of heart-healthy food tips:

F.Y.I. **Facts about heart disease and diabetes**

- 80 percent of deaths in people with diabetes are from cardiovascular disease.
- Cardiovascular disease is responsible for 75 percent of hospitalizations.
- 50 percent of people with diabetes have evidence of cardiovascular disease at the time they were diagnosed with type II diabetes.

[Am. J Cardiol 90(Suppl) s55I-62I, 2002]

THE A-Z GUIDE TO A HEALTHY HEART

An apple a day keeps the cardiologist away. Ben Franklin might not have said those exact words, but it's not such a crazy idea. In fact, in the last decade, there's been plenty of promising research about the power of foods and nutrients to keep our cardiovascular systems healthy and ward off heart disease—the number-one killer of both men and women in the United States. There are different ways that foods help decrease the risk of heart disease, including lowering blood lipids so fatty plaque is less likely to be deposited in the arteries, making components of the blood less likely to stick together, and making our arterial walls more flexible.

A-arachidonic acid—an omega-6 fatty acid: When we eat too much of the omega-6 fatty acid, arachidonic acid, some is converted to thromboxane A2 and other compounds—eicosanoids—which tend to enhance atherosclerosis by promoting vasoconstriction and platelet aggregation.

Almonds: A daily snack-size dose of almonds significantly reduced coronary heart disease risk factors in men and women with high blood cholesterol by lowering LDL cholesterol and the LDL to HDL cholesterol ratio. Higher doses of almonds also decreased lipoprotein (a) and oxidized LDL cholesterol levels.

Apples: Apples are rich in soluble fiber, the type of fiber that helps lower total serum cholesterol and LDL cholesterol. Soluble fiber also helps regulate blood sugars. One large apple (with peel) gives you over 4 grams of fiber. Just remember to eat the skin, because studies suggest that's where a lot of the food's antioxidants are found.

B-vitamins: The three B-vitamins (folate, B6, and B12) work together to reduce the level of homocysteine, which, in high levels, is thought to damage the lining of arteries, leading to heart attacks.

Beans: Beans are nutritional powerhouses and we would benefit from eating them several times a week. They are rich in fiber (especially soluble fiber), phytoestrogens, other beneficial phytochemicals that help protect the body from disease (including protease inhibitors, phytosterols, and saponins), and vitamins such as folic acid and minerals such as calcium.

Blue fruits and vegetables: Blue/purple fruits and vegetables contain anthocyanins and phenolics (among other phytochemicals and nutrients), which are being studied for their potential antioxidant and anti-aging benefits (blackberries, blueberries, purple grapes, plums, eggplant, etc.).

Canola oil: Many experts suggest switching to canola oil for cooking and baking because it is has a neutral taste and can be heated to high temperatures, not to mention it is rich in the more heart friendly, monounsaturated fats and contains more plant omega-3s than any other vegetable oil. Omega-3s are highly protective against heart disease, protecting against atherosclerosis and fatal cardiovascular events and strokes, cardiac arrhythmias, and hypertension.

Chocolate: Natural compounds in chocolate, called flavonoids, can be absorbed into the blood, and University of California, Davis, researchers have noted that there is a reduction in the tendency for platelets (part of red blood cells) to clot (similar to the effects of taking a baby aspirin) after cocoa beverages are consumed. Among the natural plant chemicals (phytochemicals) found in the cacao bean (and chocolate) are flavonoids (considered strong antioxidants). The higher-flavonoid chocolate the Davis researchers used caused some favorable relaxation or dilation of blood vessels as well.

DASH Study: In the first DASH trial, a diet rich in fruits and vegetables, low in total fat and saturated fat, plus incorporating low-fat dairy products had a positive effect on participants' blood pressures. But in the second trial, when sodium restrictions were added (along with the previous combination diet), it was even more effective in lowering blood pressure levels.

Dairy: Reduce the fat and increase the calcium and protein! When you choose lower fat dairy products, you not only get less fat and calories, you get more calcium and protein. Look at the difference it makes in milk and cheddar cheese:

- Milk (whole): 1 cup = 150 calories, 8.2 g fat, 290 mg calcium, 8.1 g protein.
- Milk (1 percent low-fat): 1 cup = 102 calories, 2.6 g fat, 300 mg calcium, 8.1 g protein.

- Cheddar Cheese (regular): 1 ounce = 114 calories, 9.4 g fat, 204 mg calcium, 7 g protein.
- Cheddar Cheese (Kraft low-fat): 1 ounce = 81 calories, 5 g fat, 253 mg calcium, 9 g protein.

Another plus: Lower fat dairy and leaner beef cuts will also contain less total fat, less saturated fat and less trans fats!

DHA (Docosahexaenoic acid): This is a powerful omega-3 fatty acid found in fish. DHA is one of the two powerful long chain omega-3 fatty acids found in fish (the other is EPA). Fish-eaters have fewer coronary heart disease events than those who seldom eat fish. The strongest epidemiological association between any fatty acid and heart disease protection is for the long chain omega-3 fatty acids in fish, one of which is DHA.

Edamame (boiled soybeans for snacking): These hip new appetizers are only a 5-minute microwave setting away. You can buy them in bags in the frozen-vegetable aisle of your supermarket. Not only is this a fun way to get soy serving, 1/2 cup of shelled beans also contains 8 grams of fiber (and only 90 calories and 2 grams fat).

Eggs (with extra omega-3 fatty acids): By feeding hens a higher omega-3 diet (from flaxseed, canola oil, etc.) they produce higher omega-3 eggs. In one study, feeding flaxseed increased the plant omega-3s in the egg yolk about 30 times and increased the level of DHA (one of the long chain omega-3s found in fish) to nearly 4 times the amount in regular eggs. When the eggs were fed to people for 4 weeks straight, the stickiness of the blood platelets decreased significantly and serum triglycerides decreased as well. Higher omega-3 eggs are being sold throughout the country under various brands, such as "Eggland's Best."

Escarole: Also known as curly endive, escarole is a great source of the antioxidant folic acid (1 cup of uncooked escarole contains 39 percent of the daily value) and a good source of vitamin A (1 cup contains 13 percent daily value) . . . all for just 8 calories!

Fiber: It's hard to believe that something we can't even digest and absorb can be so good for us. Believe it.

- Soluble fiber lowers blood cholesterol levels and helps normalize blood glucose and insulin levels (important in the prevention of cardiovascular disease and type II diabetes).
- Insoluble fiber helps move things along in the large intestine (promoting regular bowel movements and preventing constipation problems).
- Fiber-rich meals in general help little tummies—and grown up tummies for that matter—feel fuller faster (helping to prevent obesity). Meals that are higher in fiber are processed more slowly and take longer to digest and are usually large in volume but less dense with calories.

Flavonoids (a family of phytochemicals) show heart-protective effects and are considered strong antioxidants with assorted proposed heart protective effects (antioxidant, antithrombotic, anti-ischaemic, and relaxing blood vessel walls). Many population studies have shown that eating flavonoid-rich food is often associated with reduced risk of heart disease. You can find them in berries, purple grapes, and green tea. The combination of flavonoids and omega-3 fatty acids (found in fish and certain plant foods) may reduce the formation of clots, leading to heart attacks and strokes.

Folic acid (folacin): Folic acid acts as an antioxidant in the body and is thought (along with the B6 and B12), to help get your homocysteine levels back to normal (a number of studies link elevated homocysteine levels with possible risk of damage to heart arteries). The risk or need for revascularization of target lesions and of overall adverse cardiac events were reduced in one study after participants (with known coronary artery disease) took a daily dose of prescription-strength folic acid (1 mg/d), vitamin B12

(400 mg/d), and vitamin B6 (10 mg/d) for six months. A just-released study suggested that another B-vitamin, riboflavin, may interact with folic acid to also help lower homocysteine levels.

Garlic: Garlic extract containing the phytochemical allicin was tested on rats with high serum cholesterol and resulted in lower blood cholesterol, triglyceride, and blood pressure levels.

Green fruits and vegetables contain lutein and indoles (among other phytochemicals and nutrients), which have potential antioxidant and health promoting benefits (incuded are: green apples, green grapes, honeydew melon, kiwifruit, green pears, artichokes, asparagus, broccoli, brussels sprouts, bok choy, green beans, green cabbage, celery, leafy greens, leeks, green lettuce, green pepper, spinach, zucchini, and peas).

Ground flaxseed may reduce the risk for heart disease by lowering the risk of blood clots and stroke, cardiac arrythmias, reducing total cholesterol and LDL cholesterol, triglycerides, and blood pressure. Eating it whole, however, may not give the same benefits.

Halibut, herring, and other fish: "Eat fish twice a week for the most benefit" is the recommendation echoed by heart disease experts and government health agencies. Fish contains omega-3 fatty acids, which lower blood pressure and cholesterol, reducing the risk of heart disease and stroke. Salmon, tuna (even canned albacore tuna in water), trout, striped bass, mackerel, halibut, herring, sardines, shellfish, and shrimp all qualify as fish! (Pregnant women should not eat shark, swordfish, and king mackerel due to potentially high mercury levels.)

Hazelnuts have one of the highest amount of monounsaturated fats of all the nuts. One ounce of these nuts contains: 185 calories, 2 g fiber, 18.5 g fat, 1.4 g saturated fat, 14.6 g monounsaturated fat, and 1.7 g omega-6.

HDLs (good cholesterol): A new study found high levels of HDLs cut risk of stroke by 47 percent. How can we get our HDLs (good cholesterol) to work for us? Eat a diet rich in monounsaturated fats and omega-3 fatty acids as part of a lower diet, and avoid trans fats and maintain a healthy weight.

Hydrogenated and partially hydrogenated fat: A fat that has been chemically altered (made more saturated and therefore more solid) by the addition of "hydrogen" atoms. If a vegetable oil is completely saturated, or "hydrogenated," it becomes a saturated fat. When a vegetable oil is partially hydrogenated, some trans fatty acids are formed. Margarine and shortening are examples of partially hydrogenated and hydrogenated fats.

Hydrogenated vegetable oils should be limited.

Isoflavones are an important phytochemical. Many of the health benefits of soy have been attributed to the isoflavones (phytochemicals) in soybeans. A recent study on high and low isoflavone diets showed small but significant decreases in LDL cholesterol and the LDL to HDL ratio in postmenopausal women with both normal and mildly high cholesterol levels. Isoflavones are also found in apples, berries, broccoli, cabbage, carrots, citrus fruits, garlic, grapes, peppers, lettuce, strawberries, squash, tomatoes, and yams.

Japanese women: A Japanese study looked at the flavonoid and isoflavone intake of a sample of women. The results suggested that a high consumption of both of these phytochemicals by Japanese women may contribute to their low incidence of coronary heart disease compared with women in other countries. The major souce of flavonoids was onions, and of isoflavones, was tofu.

Jicama: This Mexican root vegetable is available year-round and is a refreshing addition to a vegetable platter or can be used as a fresh substitute for canned water chestnuts. One cup of crunchy jicama contributes over 5 grams of fiber, 40 percent of the daily value for vitamin C (24 mg), and 69 percent of the daily value for vitamin E (5.5 mg).

Juice (orange): One of the easiest ways to get your recommended daily intake of folic acid is to drink a glass of orange juice. A recent study on a Mediterranean population (with natural plant foods as their main source of folic acid) found evidence that dietary folic acid intake may be an independent protective factor for myocardial infarction. One cup of orange juice contains about half the daily value for folic acid.

Kale: This dark green member of the cruciferous vegetable family is as good as an antioxidant shot in the arm. One cup of cooked kale delivers 120 percent of the daily value for vitamin A, 88 percent for vitamin C, 10 percent for folic acid, and 12 percent for vitamin E. It also contributes 12 percent of the daily value for calcium, and contains 2.5 grams of fiber, and just 42 calories.

Kidney beans are not only one of the best plant sources of omega-3 fatty acids, they also give you 7 grams of fiber per 1/2 cup, along with lots of vitamins and minerals (for example, 64 percent of the daily value for folic acid and 17 percent for iron) and assorted phytochemicals.

Lignans: Lignans (phytoestrogens found in kidney beans, soybeans, lentils, navy beans, pinto beans, pears, plums, asparagus, beets, bell peppers, broccoli, carrots, cauliflower, leeks, onions, snowpeas, squash, sweet potatoes, and turnips) exhibit anti-inflammatory actions, which means they help block the pro-inflammatory actions of platelet activating factor. Lignans also have antioxidant properties and may help block the oxidation of LDL "bad" cholesterol particles, encouraging fewer of them to deposit in your arterial walls.

Lycopene: A potent antioxidant carotenoid, lycopene is a phytochemical in the carotenoid grouping with antioxidant properties and is thought to protect against the early stages of heart disease. Tomatoes and processed tomato products are the major source of lycopene in North America, although it is also found in other red fruits and vegetables (watermelons, pink grapefruits, apricots, and pink guavas).

Lp (a), Lipoprotein (a) is similar in structure to LDL "bad" cholesterol and may be a strong indicator of heart disease risk in women. LpA may worsen atherosclerosis by inhibiting your body's ability to dissolve blood clots—increasing your risk of heart attacks.

Magnesium: Abnormally low levels of magnesium in the blood are related to diabetes and high blood pressure (an increased intake of magnesium might lower blood pressure). Recently a study revealed that there is also a strong relationship between decreased levels of blood magnesium and metabolic syndrome (metabolic syndrome was defined as people with two or more of the following: hyperglycemia, high blood pressure, elevated blood lipids, and obesity). Magnesium is found in nuts and beans; certain leafy green vegetables, such as broccoli and spinach; potatoes; and smaller amounts in whole grain foods, meats, seafood, and milk.

Margarine (Smart Balance): Smart Balance margarine is one of the only margarines that doesn't use hydrogenated oils and therefore doesn't contain trans fatty acids. It uses a blend of vegetables oils (soy, palm, canola, and olive) to produce a balance of saturated, monounsaturated, and polyunsaturated fat.

McDonald's (Filet-O-Fish): If you see the calories and fat grams listed for the McDonald's Filet-O-Fish sandwich, you would think most of the fat is coming from the fried fish filet. Guess again—it's the sauce. Take the tartar sauce off the fish sandwich and the calories go from 470 to 325 and fat grams go from 26 to 10.

Mediterranean olive oil: People in the Mediterranean region have been studied lately because they have surprisingly low rates of heart disease and the use of olive oil is a key characteristic of their cuisine (which also includes abundant seafood, fruits, vegetables, and nuts). The majority of fatty acids in olive oil are the more beneficial monounsaturated fats. Olive oil also contains some of the potentially protective phytochemicals found in olives.

Nectarines: Not to be mistaken for a fuzzless peach, nectarines have been a variety of fruit for around 2,000 years. Like peaches, though, nectarines are a good source of antioxidants. One nectarine brings you 13 percent of the daily value for vitamin A (as a carotene), 12 percent of the daily value for vitamin C (7.5 mg), and 15 percent of the daily value for vitamin E (1.2 mg), along with 2 grams of fiber and 66 calories.

Nuts: The frequency of nut consumption has been found to be protective against coronary heart disease (CHD) risk in five epidemiological studies. Nut-rich diets have been shown to lower serum cholesterol and the magnitude of the CHD risk reduction is greater than might be explained by changes in blood lipids alone.

Some nuts contain monounsaturated fats that, when substituted for other fatty foods, can lower "bad" LDL cholesterol and reduce the risk of heart disease. In addition to unsaturated fats, nuts are high in protein, dietary fiber, tocopherols (vitamin E), magnesium, copper, several phytosterols, bioflavonoids, and other important phytochemicals.

Oats: One of the first health claims allowed on food labels was the claim for the soluble fiber in oats and oat bran in cardiovascular risk management. The consumption of about 25 grams a day of oat-containing foods can reduce the risk of heart disease.

Omega-3 fatty acids (found in fish and some plant foods) appear to provide protection against atherosclerosis and fatal cardiovascular events and strokes, cardiac arrhythmias, and hypertension. Omega-3s from fish lower triglyceride levels and raise HDL "good" cholesterol.

The onion and garlic family: One group of phytochemicals in raw onion and garlic juice, which includes thiosulfinates and allicin, has demonstrated that they help platelets keep from sticking together (similar to the effects of the same concentration of aspirin). Another study on rats suggested these compounds can also encourage relaxation of the pulmonary arteries.

Oranges and other citrus fruits boost our intake of vitamin C, folic acid, potassium, and soluble fiber and a host of active phytochemicals such as polyphenols, which act as strong antioxidants and could reduce the incidence and severity of heart disease. According to a recent analysis, polyphenols accounted for 84 percent of the antioxidant quality in orange juice.

Plant omega-3s: Substituting plant omega-3s for saturated fat in the diet enhances the blood cholesterol-lowering benefits of the omega-3s. One study found that as the plant omega-3 content of blood cholesterol esters and phospholipids went up, the risk of stroke went down. The study also calculated that each standard deviation increase in plant omega-3s (alpha-linolenic acid) was associated with a 30-percent reduction in stroke risk.

Plant stanol and sterol spreads: Benecol and Take Control are two brands of stanol- and sterol-enhanced spreads that can be used in place of butter or margarine. Daily intakes of 2 to 3 grams can lower LDL cholesterol by 10 to 15 percent. The plant stanols and sterols are similar to cholesterol and when they are in the intestine, they lower the absorption of cholesterol there.

Prospective trials: What have they taught us about diet and heart disease? Large prospective trials show that groups of people who experience the fewest cases of heart disease have a general pattern of eating that is rich in fish, polyunsaturated fatty acids, whole grain cereals, fruits and vegetables, and low-fat dairy foods; and low in saturated fat from dairy fat, meat fat, and fried foods.

Produce: Eating your fruits and vegetables, particularly vitamin C-rich fruits and vegetables and green leafy vegetables, appears to have a protective effect against heart disease, according to a large Harvard study. Including one more serving of fruits and vegetables per day was associated with a 4-percent lower risk for coronary heart disease.

Psyllium is high in soluble fiber. You'll find some of your best soluble fiber sources are beans, oats, legumes, psyllium, barley, prunes, guava, flaxseed, and pectin. Many of the over-the-counter fiber supplements (that you mix with water and drink) use ground psyllium seed.

Quercetin: A key phytochemical in the flavonol grouping, studies have shown that as intake of quercetin increases, mortality from coronary heart disease decreases. The results of one particular study also suggest that quercetin might be benefiting the body, in part, through the stabilization of plaque.

Raspberries: Fiber-packed raspberries give you 5 grams of fiber in each cup, antioxidants, folic acid (18 percent of the daily value), and vitamin C (51 percent of the daily value).

Red fruits and vegetables (red apples, tomatoes, cherries, cranberries, red grapes, red pears, raspberries, strawberries, red cabbage, red peppers, red potatoes, and rhubarb) contain lycopene and anthocyanins (among other phytochemicals and nutrients), which are being studied for their health-promoting properties.

Restaurants and fast food: Americans need to eat out less or, at the very least, make healthier choices when they are eating out. Consumption of food prepared away from home increased from 18 percent to 32 percent of total calories between 1977–78 and 1994–96. All this "away food" has not only been shown to contain more calories, total fat, and saturated fat per eating occasion, but it also contains less fiber (on a per-calorie basis) than food prepared at home.

Saturated fat: Don't let the information you have read about the dangers of trans fats distract you from the importance of also reducing saturated fats in our daily diet. Americans eat far more saturated fat than trans fat. Reducing both fats is vital to our health.

Selenium: Selenium deficiency in humans has been implicated in the etiology of heart disease, but there is still only limited evidence. However, stay tuned—intervention studies are under way to assess the benefits of selenium (a key antioxidant) supplements in the prevention of atherosclerosis.

Soy, tofu, and other soy foods may help protect our heart and arteries by making the fats in our blood less damaging and plaque less likely to form.

Strawberries are rich in antioxidants. One cup of sliced strawberries contains 16 percent of the daily value for folic acid, and 157 percent for vitamin C, plus 2.5 grams of fiber. A recent study where rats were fed large amounts of strawberries found that the older rats started acting physically and mentally younger than their years.

Tea: Several population studies have shown that a higher tea intake is associated with a lower incidence of heart disease, but other studies found no protective effect. It seems that one explanation could be (and this was looked at further in a number of studies) that the quercetin phytochemical in tea is more available to/absorbable for women than for men. This may be due to hormones and the gastrointestinal tract's natural bacteria. This "female effect" was demonstrated in several studies.

Tomatoes are loaded with lycopene, not to mention vitamin C and a host of other vitamins and phytochemicals. The suggested daily intake of lycopene is 35 mg, which you can meet by drinking two glasses of tomato juice or through a combination of tomato products. Recent studies have demonstrated that the heat processing of tomatoes and tomato products makes the lycopene in the product more available to the body.

Trans fats should be limited. Health-wise, trans fatty acids' damaging effects are akin to those of saturated fat, except trans fats offer a double whammy to your blood lipid profile. In addition to increasing your bad cholesterol (LDL) and saturated fat levels, trans fats also decrease your "good cholesterol" (HDL) levels at the same time. This is one of the reasons many researchers consider trans fats to be a bigger enemy than saturated fats.

Consumption of trans fats is related to increased risk of coronary heart disease:

- Trans fats raise blood levels of LDL "bad" cholesterol (low-density lipoproteins).
- Trans fats lower HDL "good" cholesterol (high-density lipoproteins).
- Trans fats also elevate lipoprotein (see definition below).
- Trans fats may help inflame and stiffen the arteries (not a good thing).

Umbelliferous vegetables (a botanical grouping), such as carrots and celery, contain varying amounts of pro-vitamin A and other important carotenoid phytochemicals. One carrot contains 2025 RE of carotene/vitamin A (253 percent of the daily value). An Italian study found that as the consumption of certain foods (such as fish, carrots, and green vegetables) increased, the risk of heart attack decreased.

Unsaturated fats: When saturated or trans fats are replaced with unsaturated fats (monounsaturated fats or omega-6 polyunsaturated fats from vegetable oils) LDL "bad" cholesterol decreases and the LDL to HDL "good" cholesterol ratio also decreases, according to a recent study.

Vegetable oils: The following are commonly used vegetable oils that have very high amounts of omega-6 fatty acids and very low amounts of omega-3 fatty acids, or are extraordinarily high in saturated fat (tropical oils) and would be best replaced, when possible, with a high monounsaturated fat vegetable oil (olive oil and canola oil) or higher omega-3 oil (canola):

- Tropical oils (palm kernel oil, coconut oil, palm oil).
- Corn oil.
- Safflower oil.
- Cottonseed oil.
- Sunflower oil.

Vegetarian entrées: Try them sometime, you might like them! Favorable cardiovascular effects have been reported with vegetarian and semi-vegetarian diets. This may be because vegetarian meals tend to be higher in fruits and vegetables and fiber and lower in saturated fat.

Viscous (soluble) fiber: Viscous or gelatinous fiber (soluble) interferes with bile acid absorption from the lower end of the small intestines, which means less bile acid is reabsorbed and recycled. This causes more LDL or "bad" cholesterol to be removed from the blood and converted into new bile acids to replace those lost in the stool. There is even evidence that the presence of some viscous fibers in the intestines may decrease cholesterol synthesis—so you're beating cholesterol coming and going, so to speak. Your best food sources of soluble fiber are oats and oat bran, barley, beans, psyllium seed products, apples, bananas, citrus fruits, carrots, green beans, and ground flaxseed.

Vitamin C: Eating your fruits and vegetables, particularly green leafy vegetables and vitamin C-rich fruits and vegetables, appears to have a protective effect against heart disease, according to a large Harvard study. Including one more serving of fruits and vegetables per day was associated with a 4-percent lower risk for coronary heart disease.

Walnuts: Intervention trials have demonstrated that walnuts (as part of a heart-healthy diet) decrease blood cholesterol levels. In addition to having the highest amount of plant omega-3s of any of the nuts, walnuts also have phytochemicals such as polyphenols, omega-6 fatty acids, folic acid, and fiber. One ounce of black walnuts contains: 170 calories, 1 g fiber, 16 g fat, 1 g saturated fat, 3.6 g monounsaturated fat, and .9 g omega-3 fatty acids.

Whole grains: Switch from refined grains to whole grains whenever possible! The phytochemicals and cereal fiber in whole grains help reduce the risk of heart disease in both men and women. Whole grains are also digested more slowly than refined grains, and appear to help increase the body's sensitivity to insulin. A study of nearly 3,000 middle-aged adults found that eating whole-grain foods was associated with improved insulin sensitivity and lower LDL "bad" cholesterol levels. When refined rice was replaced with whole grain and legume powder as a source of the carbohydrate in the meal, a Korean study showed beneficial effects on glucose and insulin levels as well as homocysteine concentrations and lipid peroxidation in patients with coronary artery disease.

Whole-wheat tortillas: There are several brands of whole-wheat tortillas in supermarkets near you. The one made by the Tortilla Factory contains whole wheat flour, oat fiber, soybean flour and canola oil, and has 9 grams of fiber (2 grams fat: 1 gram polyunsaturated and 1 gram monounsaturated) and only 60 calories!

Whopper: It's amazing how the calories and fat grams go down when you "undress" certain fast food sandwiches. Burger King's Whopper with cheese and mayonnaise adds up to 795 calories and 53 grams of fat, compared to the Whopper with cheese but without mayonnaise, which totals 695 calories and 36 grams of fat. Go all the way and cut out the cheese and the mayo and it gets down to 605 calories and 28 grams of fat.

Syndrome X: One third of middle-aged Americans have syndrome X (also known as metabolic syndrome) and many have no idea that they do. Metabolic syndrome is a cluster of health problems (large tummy, high blood sugar, lower than average HDL "good" cholesterol, high triglycerides, and high blood pressure) caused by a combination of genes and lifestyle factors (eating too much and not exercising enough).

Yellow/orange fruits and vegetables contain varying amounts of all sorts of antioxidants, such as vitamin C, as well as phytochemicals such as carotenoids and bioflavonoids (both of which are being studied for their health promoting potential). Produce in this group includes apricots, cantaloupe, grapefruit, lemons, mangoes, nectarines, oranges, papayas, peaches, persimmons, butternut squash, carrots, and sweet potatoes.

Yogurt: One serving of yogurt contains almost as much calcium as you would get in a calcium supplement. A recent study found that people with controlled high blood pressure have a higher calcium intake than non-controlled. But calcium is not the only thing yogurt has going for it. A daily yogurt serving containing lactobacillus acidophilus (human origin), as revealed in two clinical studies, led to a small reduction in serum cholesterol concentration, which would translate to a potential of reducing risk for coronary heart disease by 6 to 10 percent. One cup of low-fat fruit yogurt contains 47 percent of the daily value of calcium, 35 percent of B2, 9 percent of B1, 57 percent of B12, 13 percent of folic acid, 13 percent of magnesium, 24 percent of potassium, 10 percent of selenium, and 15 percent of zinc.

Zucchini: A popular vegetable, 1 cup of cooked zucchini adds up to only 29 calories but is loaded with nutrients: 2.5 grams fiber, 9 percent of the daily value of vitamin B6, 17 percent of folic acid, 14 percent of vitamin C, 14 percent of magnesium, and 23 percent of potassium.

Chapter 4

The 10 Food Steps to Freedom

T rue, you need to work out an individualized eating plan with your dietitian or certified diabetes educator because what works best to normalize your blood sugars may be different for someone else. But there are 10 things all people with type II diabetes can do to improve their health, reduce their risk of heart disease and other health risks, and to make normal blood sugars more likely. That's what you will find here in the 10 Food Steps to Freedom.

I'd better come clean right from the get-go though—two of the 10 "food" steps to freedom don't really involve food. One is monitoring your blood sugar levels and the other is regular exercise. They both help bring you food freedom. Monitoring blood sugars is the best way to understand how certain meals and snacks affect your personal blood sugars—a pivotal tool in helping fine-tune your eating plan. Exercise acts like insulin in the body and can quite possibly make normal blood sugars easier to achieve, which will give you a little more freedom in the food department. Following these 10 steps will bring you one giant step closer to feeling better, having normal blood sugars, and living a longer, healthier life.

Step #1: Make fiber a part of almost every meal

Fiber is the part in plant foods that humans can't digest. Because we can't digest it, it makes it all the way through the mouth to the stomach and then through the small and large intestines (without being absorbed) and out the other end. But even though it isn't absorbed, it does all sorts of great stuff for our bodies.

There are two types of fiber. There is the kind that doesn't dissolve in water (called insoluble fiber), which contributes "roughage" or "bulk" to our intestinal tract. It acts like a scrubber, pushing food along and helping to clean the intestinal wall as it passes through. This is the type of fiber that is thought to help treat and prevent diverticulosis (when small pouches form in the colon wall and can become infected) and linked to reducing the risk of constipation and colon cancer. It is possible that the fiber latches onto potential carcinogens (cancer-causing agents) within the intestines and carries them out of the body.

The other type of fiber is particularly important if you have type II diabetes—soluble fiber. Soluble fiber is different from the other type of fiber because it dissolves in water and becomes almost gel-like. Soluble fiber does appear to lower total serum cholesterol and LDL cholesterol levels (the higher your cholesterol levels, the more it will help lower it). It also helps regulate blood sugars. Because soluble fiber helps regulate blood sugars, high fiber diets have been reported to:

- Lower postprandial (after meals) blood sugar. (It may even improve glucose control in the meals immediately following.)
- Decrease glucose in the urine (because it helps lower blood sugars).

- Decrease insulin needs and increase tissue sensitivity to insulin.
- Reduce levels of atherosclerosis-promoting blood lipids.

It's the soluble fiber in particular that may help lessen the potential increase in blood triglycerides and other blood fats seen in some diabetics on a high carbohydrate diet.

One study with type II people showed that a high-fiber eating plan reduced insulin requirements by 75 percent. Some people were able to get off insulin completely. There is one catch—soluble fiber helps lower your glucose level after meals, and to a lesser extent your wake-up glucose reading (fasting glucose). But this is still super helpful because we spend most of our 24-hour day in a postmeal state, right? How much fiber are we talking about? A stiff daily dose of about 30 grams of fiber.

How much fiber do we need to get our heart disease prevention benefits? About the same amount. In one study, men who ate more than 25 grams of fiber per day reduced their risk of heart disease by 36 percent, compared to men who ate less than 15 grams of fiber daily. Does this sound impossible? With the right tips and recipes, and maybe a small hill of beans, some of us can hit this mark on most days.

How does soluble fiber work its magic?

The fiber slows down the absorption of other nutrients eaten at the same meal, including carbohydrates. This slowing down may help prevent peaks and valleys in your blood sugars. (It has also been suggested that higher fiber meals improve your body sensitivity to insulin, so it may reduce the insulin requirements in insulin-treated type II diabetics.)

As it passes through the intestines, soluble fiber holds on to anything it can and carries it out of the body. One of the things we know it holds on to is bile (digestive juices that the body produces using cholesterol from the body), so our body has to keep making more bile—using more cholesterol. This reduces blood cholesterol levels. Every body responds differently, but for some people, combining soluble fiber with a low-fat eating plan can mean serum cholesterol reductions of 50 points or more.

There is also some evidence that soluble fiber can slow the liver's manufacture of cholesterol as well as change LDL particles so they are larger and less dense and dangerous to our arteries. Soluble fiber may also hold on to some fats and carbohydrate from the food we just ate along with the soluble fiber—"eliminating" it before it is absorbed.

Getting fiber at almost every meal

The problem is the typical American diet is anything but high in fiber. "White" grain is the American mode of operation—we eat a muffin or bagel made with white flour in the morning, have our hamburger on a white bun, then have white rice with our dinner. The more refined or "whiter" the grain-based food, the lower the fiber.

To get some fiber into almost every meal takes effort. Start by:

- Eating plenty of fruits and vegetables. Just eating five servings a day of fruits and vegetables (something we should do anyway) will get you to about 5 grams of soluble fiber. See Step #6 on page 95 for more on fruits and vegetables.

- Include some beans and bean products often (1/2 cup of cooked beans will add about 2 grams of soluble fiber to your day).

- Switch to less refined grains (whole grain breads and cereals, oats, brown and wild rice, barley, etc.) whenever possible.

Personally I have come to enjoy my daily fruits and vegetables. I crave beans and tofu frequently, and I don't even mind whole grain breads or using part whole wheat flour in my muffins. But I don't think I will ever get used to whole wheat pasta. That's where I personally draw the line. I do, however, buy only 100-percent semolina flour pasta (which seems to have a lower blood glucose effect compared to other pastas for many people). The point is, each of us is going to draw the line in different places. Some of you might find white rice nonnegotiable while others insist on sourdough, French, or white bread. And that's okay. Just switch where you can. But if you are going to eat good old "white" bread, at least buy brands that have added soluble fiber sources (malted barley flour, soy fiber, and oat fiber) and other nutrients (calcium and folic acid).

Where can you find soluble fiber?

Most plant foods contain some insoluble fiber and some soluble fiber. About one-quarter to one-third of the total amount of fiber in plants is the soluble type—but some plant foods have more than others. The following foods are some of the richest sources of soluble fiber.

Beans. One-half cup cooked kidney beans, cranberry beans, butterbeans, canned baked beans, blackbeans, navy beans, lentils, pinto beans, great northern beans, chick peas or garbanzo, split peas, and lima beans. Some of the soluble fiber dissolves in the liquid of canned beans so if you are making a soup or stew, just stir the liquid in.

Oats and oat bran. One-half cup dry oat bran contributes 3 grams of soluble fiber, and 1 cup of cooked oatmeal contains about 2 grams of soluble fiber. One packet of instant oatmeal contributes 1 gram of soluble fiber.

Barley. This grain has been enjoyed in other parts of the world for hundreds of years. In America, you sometimes find it in soups. Even pearl barley, which has been milled, still contributes 1.8 grams of soluble fiber per 3/4-cup cooked serving.

Some fruits. Apples; mango; plums; kiwi; pears; blackberries; strawberries; raspberries; peaches; citrus fruits, including oranges and grapefruits (you'll get the most soluble fiber if you include the "pulp" and membranes dividing the fruit into sections); dried fruits including dried apricots, prunes, and figs.

Some vegetables. Artichokes, celery root, sweet potato, parsnip, turnip, acorn squash, potato with skin, brussels sprouts, cabbage, green peas, broccoli, carrots, french-style green beans, cauliflower, asparagus, and beets.

Psyllium seed products. One rounded kitchen teaspoon of most psyllium products will give you about 3 grams of soluble fiber.

F.Y.I. Psyllium isn't silly, it means business

Psyllium fiber, in combination with a low-fat diet, has been shown to reduce after-meal blood glucose levels. Soluble fiber, in general, has been shown to reduce total cholesterol and LDL-cholesterol levels (all good things).

An eight-week study with psyllium fiber (two packets of Metamucil—5.1 grams psyllium fiber per packet) showed some encouraging results:

- Serum LDL-cholesterol levels decreased 4.9 percent.
- All-day, after-meal serum glucose levels declined 4.2 percent with after-lunch serum glucose reading declining by 6.5 percent.

[Am J Clin Nutr 70: 146-173. 1999]

Give it time and lots of water

Most people's bodies seem to adjust to more fiber in their diet within about six weeks. While your body is "adjusting" you may notice a little uninvited gas. To minimize the uninvited side effects (diarrhea, abdominal pain, and flatulence) increase your fiber slowly and drink plenty of water (which you should be doing anyway). Soluble fiber, especially, absorbs water like a sponge, so drink up (only decaf, nonalcoholic beverages count toward the recommended eight glasses of water a day).

You can also try Beano pills or drops (you find them in your local drugstore), which contain an enzyme that, when taken along with beans, cabbage, broccoli, and other vegetables, helps reduce the side effects. If you are using dry beans, don't cook the beans in the soaking liquid because the gas-producing sugars leach into the water. Some people do find there are some foods you simply cannot adjust to, like certain beans or cabbage. For a handful of great bean recipes, see Chapter 5. For lists of higher fiber cereals and convenience products, see Chapter 6.

The high fiber bonus for calorie watchers

Both fiber types help us feel fuller faster when they are part of the meal—discouraging overeating. When people eat meals higher in fiber, they tend to eat less. One study found that people ate smaller lunches after eating high fiber breakfasts. Why? Fiber lowers insulin and insulin helps stimulate your appetite. And fiber seems to help make you feel full.

There is also some evidence that fiber can help cut calories by blocking the digestion of some of the fat, protein, or carbohydrates eaten at the same time. Either way, it's a good thing if you are overweight.

What's the Quickest Way to 30 Grams of Fiber?

1. Get at least 5 servings of fruits and vegetables every day.

- Add fruit in the morning, fruit as a snack (dried fruits like dried apricots, prunes, and figs are particularly high in soluble fiber), and fruit as or with dessert.

- If you drink orange or grapefruit juice, opt for the kind "with pulp" to boost your soluble fiber.

- Include a vegetable with lunch, have raw vegetables as an afternoon snack or pre-dinner appetizer, then enjoy vegetables with dinner.

2. Include a serving of beans several times a week.

- Research is showing that a diet high in legumes (beans and peas) somehow improves all aspects of diabetes control (lowered blood sugars and improved blood lipid levels).

3. Include a high fiber cereal almost every day at breakfast or as a snack.

- Have oatmeal (or another high oat-bran food) often for breakfast, or as an evening snack.

- Switch to "whole" grains when possible such as brown or wild rice and whole wheat or whole grain bread. Use part whole wheat flour when making breads or muffins at home.

4. Perhaps for some, include a serving of a high-fiber supplement.

- Ground flaxseed (see Step #8 on page 101 for more about flaxseed).

- Bran Buds combines some less concentrated psyllium with wheat.

- About a tablespoon of 100-percent psyllium supplement with no chemical stimulants taken with a meal once a day. But make sure you are drinking your obligatory eight glasses of water a day and consult your doctor, dietitian, or diabetes educator first! A small number of people have an allergic reaction to it and it can also alter the absorption of other medications you may be taking. Psyllium in powdered form is recommended by one researcher who used Sugar-Free Orange Metamucil in a study. You mix the tablespoon of the powder with juice, cereals, soups, etc. But eat or drink the mixture soon. If you don't, you'll need a spoon not a straw (soluble fiber forms a gel remember?).

Keep in mind, researchers don't know as much as they would like about the safety and value of fiber supplements taken for a long period of time and that the supplements do not include the other health promoting nutrients that foods high in fiber contribute.

F.Y.I. **Beans for Lunch**

Eating beans produces a slow rise in blood sugars. The "gel" formed in the intestines makes the passage of glucose from food into the cells go in slow motion. Lunch is a very strategic time to eat beans because it will help pace your glucose absorption from food. It will keep insulin levels low, which may prevent overeating. I did notice when I was pregnant that the only lunch that would keep me from becoming absolutely ravenous midafternoon was a bean burrito.

Step #2: Count carbohydrates

Every now and then, count your carbohydrates to make sure you are hitting your desired amounts per meal/snack (and compare to your blood sugars).

It isn't that carbohydrates are bad. It's just that you need to know what amount of carbohydrates your body can tolerate (at different times of the day) given your body, medication, and exercise schedule.

Having to count anything every day gets tiresome fast. Having to write down what you eat can't help but make you feel as though you are being punished. But the truth is writing all this stuff down is one of the best ways to manage your diabetes. Keeping track of the food you eat and how your body reacted to it will help you understand what you can do better next time. It can pinpoint your particular trouble spots and your best strategies to combat them.

For example, if you find your blood sugar tends to get too high after you eat pizza, you can try eliminating the fatty meat toppings, eating one slice less, and having some green salad with vegetables and kidney beans instead. Will this lower your blood sugar response to pizza? Take your blood sugar 1 1/2 hours later and find out.

The act of keeping a food/blood sugar journal helps many people reduce their total calories. This is an added bonus to people with diabetes who are also trying to trim off a few extra pounds. I know it's hard, but try to think positively about keeping your food/blood sugar diary. Once you figure out what works best for your body, and your blood sugars become consistently normal, you won't have to keep your food diary every single day. It's a good idea to check in every once in a while though, especially if your blood sugars begin to change.

Most of the commercial food diaries available leave a space only to tabulate grams of carbohydrates. I designed the following A Day at a Glance chart on page 86 to help you tabulate grams of carbohydrate plus grams of fat and fiber. Knowing the grams of fat and fiber helps complete the picture. You might find that it's the really high fat meals that cause you trouble or you might find that a certain amount of fat grams seems to help normalize your blood sugars. You might discover that your blood sugars are better when your meal/snack contains a high fiber food.

A Day at a Glance includes a space to record how hungry you were when you ate. There is a space to record your blood sugar, your medication, and the minutes you exercised and when. All this information will help your dietitian or diabetes educator fine-tune your eating plan.

Step #3: Emphasize heart protective fats

Emphasize heart protective fats (monounsaturated fats and omega-3 fatty acids) and count fat grams for the right balance in your meals/snacks.

You might think food fat is food fat. But there are actually three types of fats in food—saturated fatty acids, polyunsaturated fatty acids, and monounsaturated fatty acids. One of them is better for you than the others. The monounsaturated fats do not seem to promote heart disease, plaquing in the arteries, and cancer, as the saturated fats and some of the polyunsaturated fats appear to. It's a no-brainer, then, to start using and eating more monounsaturated fats and definitely less saturated fat.

A Day at a Glance

Blood Sugar Measurements

6 a.m.   8 a.m.   10 a.m.   12 p.m.   2 p.m.   4 p.m.   6 p.m.   8 p.m.

Insulin or Oral Measurements
(record units or number of tablets taken at what times)

6 a.m.   8 a.m.   10 a.m.   12 p.m.   2 p.m.   4 p.m.   6 p.m.   8 p.m.

Activity (minutes)

6 a.m.   8 a.m.   10 a.m.   12 p.m.   2 p.m.   4 p.m.   6 p.m.   8 p.m.

Meals/Snacks   Day:_____ Date: ___/___/___

meal/snack	carbs	fat	fiber	hunger level

meal/snack	carbs	fat	fiber	hunger level

meal/snack	carbs	fat	fiber	hunger level

meal/snack	carbs	fat	fiber	hunger level

(*Hunger level: 4=very hungry, 3=moderately hungry,
2=somewhat hungry, 1=not really hungry)

There are basically two common oils that both contain mostly monounsaturated fats—canola oil and olive oil. They each offer additional and different health benefits (you'll find out what those are in the following sections) so I personally use both.

There are certain recipes or foods that I eat that require butter, but only if it is truly the best type of fat for that particular food. Even then, I will use the least amount I can. When I can, I switch to canola or olive oil or canola margarine. In most sautéing circumstances, I can use canola or olive oil. In many baking recipes, such as some cakes, muffins, even pie crust, I can switch to canola oil. If the cookie or cake recipe calls for creaming the shortening or butter with sugar, then usually I can use my favorite margarine, which contains a lot less butter than the recipe calls for. See Chapter 5 for more information.

Canola oil

You may have heard that canola is a "good" fat—that it contains mostly monounsaturated fat. You may have even heard that it is one of the few plant sources of omega-3 fatty acids. But how much would you need, to get a potentially beneficial dose of omega-3 fatty acids? I asked researchers at Best Foods, which makes Mazola's canola oil, to send me the actual fatty acid breakdown for one tablespoon of canola oil. I was delighted to find that just one tablespoon contained about 1.5 grams omega-3 fatty acids (about the same amount found in 3 1/2 ounces of cooked salmon). A tablespoon also contains 9 grams of omega-9 fatty acids (oleic acid, a monounsaturated fat that may reduce the development of breast carcinomas) and 7 milligrams of mixed tocopherols (a group of antioxidants that includes vitamin E, also known as alpha-tocopherol).

Canola oil has a neutral flavor and can be heated to high temperatures, so I like to use canola oil in baking and frying recipes.

Olive Oil

The people in the Mediterranean region have been studied lately because they have surprisingly low rates of heart disease, yet their typical diet is not terribly low in fat. Their cuisine includes abundant seafood, use of olives and olive oil, fruits, vegetables, and nuts. We now know that all of those foods have health benefits for our body—including olive oil.

Olive oil does not contain omega-3 fatty acids like canola oil, but the majority of fatty acids in olive oil are still the more beneficial monounsaturated fats; 56 to 83 percent of the fatty acids in olive oil are specifically oleic acid (an up-and-coming omega-9 fatty acid). Canola oil contributes more vitamin E than olive oil, but there is something that olive oil adds to your diet that canola oil doesn't—potentially protective phytochemicals found in olives.

Olive oil has a marvelous distinctive range of possible flavors, ranging from peppery to pungent, so I like to use olive oil in my Italian recipes, cold salad recipes, marinades, and vinaigrettes.

Why Count Fat Grams?

It is helpful to count fat grams because the issue of food fat for most people with type II diabetes can be a little tricky. You want enough fat to help balance carbohydrates, but not too much. The only way to know what level of fat grams works best for you at what time of day, is to count them every now and then. Take a look at your food diary and see what level of fat tends to produce better blood sugars at certain times of day.

Everybody is different but most people with type II diabetes handle carbohydrates better when they are eaten alongside some protein and fat. Fat helps lower the blood glucose response of the other foods it is eaten with. So "some"

F.Y.I. Omega-3 fatty acids

Researchers are still trying to find out as much as they can about omega-3 fatty acids. So far it looks like a win-win situation. Omega-3 fatty acids have been linked to lowering both blood pressure and serum triglyceride levels, preventing blood clots and they may even help increase HDL (good) cholesterol levels. They have also been shown to slow or prevent cancerous tumor growth as well as reduce symptoms of inflammatory diseases such as rhuematoid arthritis. The two particular cancers that omega-3s may help prevent are colon and possibly breast cancer.

Omega-3 fatty acids can be found in all sorts of fish—the fattier the better. My personal favorite fish sources are salmon, albacore tuna canned in spring water, striped bass, and pacific halibut, but you can also find them in anchovies, sardines, herring, bluefish, mackerel, mullet, and shark.

Some plant foods contain alpha-linolenic acid, which the body can partially convert to an omega-3 fatty acid. You will find alpha-linolenic acid in walnuts, walnut oil, flaxseed, rapeseed (used to make canola oil), soybeans, spinach, and mustard greens.

fat is definitely a good thing—especially if it is a rich in the more protective type of fats (monounsaturated fat, omega-3, and omega-9 fatty acids). What we are really talking about is a balancing act—pairing your carbohydrate-rich foods (breads, grains, starches, fruits, sweets, etc.) with foods that contribute some protein and fat.

It's a good idea, when you are trying to figure out which foods and food combinations you do best with, to count fat grams along with carbohydrate grams. For many people with type II diabetes, some fat helps, but meals that are too high in fat (especially highly saturated fat and animal fats) can have terrible consequences on after-meal blood sugars. In some people, meals high in animal fats make the body very resistant to insulin. Meals such as sausage and eggs breakfast or your typical pepperoni and sausage pizza can be blood glucose nightmares to many.

What this means in food terms is that we need to:

- Switch to using olive oil and canola oil (instead of other vegetable oils) when possible.
- Eat more fish.
- Eat less animal fat by choosing leaner meats and lower fat dairy products and by eating plant protein (from soy, beans, and vegetables) instead of animal protein sometimes.
- Limit foods that contain high amounts of hydrogenated and partially hydrogenated oils. (The hydrogenation process produces trans fatty acids, which are as damaging, if not more damaging, to our hearts and arteries than saturated fat.)
- You will need to figure out what to do about butter or margarine. There are some better tasting tub margarines that list liquid canola oil or olive oil as the first ingredient. If you use butter, fine. Just use less and use canola oil or olive oil in cooking instead when you can.

Cooking with the right fats

If a recipe calls for vegetable oil, just use canola oil. If it calls for vegetable oil and you think the flavor of olive oil would complement the dish and the oil wouldn't be heated to a high temperature (olive oil starts smoking and breaking down at higher temperatures), then you can even use olive oil instead. But what about the recipes that call for shortening, stick butter, or margarine? That gets a little trickier.

If you are using a lower fat recipe from the start, that helps, because whatever fat you are using is at least being added in smaller amounts. (Check out a few of my cookbooks for some great reduced fat recipes, or my national column called "The Recipe Doctor.")

Sometimes I still use butter because that truly is the best fat for that recipe. I just cut it down as far as I can (substituting in other high flavor/high moisture ingredients). But if butter isn't that essential to the recipe and your original recipe calls for beating the butter, margarine, or shortening in a mixer, usually with sugar then eggs, you can switch to a margarine with liquid canola oil as the first ingredient. Sometimes you can get away with beating part canola oil and part fat-free cream cheese or sour cream in place of the original fat. If you are just sautéing something in a pan, you can easily switch to canola or olive oil and you can probably use less than in the original recipe, especially if you are using nonstick pans.

Start collecting recipes your family likes that call for olive or canola oil. I made up a reduced fat pie crust recipe that uses canola oil. I now use salad dressings that contain canola or olive oil for my vinaigrette-dependent recipes (such as green salad and pasta salad). These are the kinds of changes you can start making right now.

Step #4: Try to keep saturated fat and cholesterol low

If monounsaturated fat is now "in," then saturated fat is definitely "out." You'd be hard-pressed to find someone who doesn't know that saturated fat is something Americans need to eat less of. High amounts of saturated fat are clearly associated with heart disease. More specifically, saturated fat has been shown to raise bad cholesterol (LDL) and triglycerides in the blood. Obviously, eating less saturated fat is good, solid advice. Giving that advice is easy, following it is the tough part—especially here in the United States. Saturated fat is synonymous with typical American food. It's in hamburgers and french fries, pizza, hot dogs, and apple pie for goodness' sake.

It doesn't matter whether you find your blood sugars improve with a low or moderate fat eating plan. Either way, saturated fat and food cholesterol need to be low. Cholesterol should be limited to 300 milligrams or less a day, and saturated fat is supposed to contribute no more than 10 percent of the total calories.

Saturated fat sources

The biggest contributor of saturated fat and cholesterol in the American diet is the meat group, which includes beef, processed meats, eggs, poultry, and other meats. In general, if you choose leaner meats (lower in fat), use egg substitute in place of half the eggs (a good rule of thumb), and take the skin off poultry, you will lower the amount of saturated fat and cholesterol.

The runner-up to meat is the milk group (includes cream and cheese)—the second largest saturated fat contributor. Select lower-fat dairy options and you are guaranteed less saturated fat and cholesterol.

Saturated fat is found in other animal fats too, such as butter, ice cream, lard, bacon, anything made with coconut and palm oil, and vegetables oils that have been "hydrogenated," as is the case with stick margarine and shortening. Many of the packaged foods we buy, such as crackers, cookies, snack foods, frozen fried foods, and pastries contain hydrogenated oils.

Where to cut cholesterol

Plant foods do not contain cholesterol. So we find cholesterol in animal foods. Where you find high amounts of fat in animals and animal products, generally cholesterol isn't far behind. Food sources highest in cholesterol are egg yolks, organ meats (especially liver), whole-fat dairy products, and higher fat meats. There are a few fish sources that are a bit higher in cholesterol, such as shrimp and squid. But they are low in fat and saturated fat—so I wouldn't worry too much about the occasional shrimp cocktail or calamari you enjoy in restaurants.

Avoiding organ meats is the easy part. Buying skin-less chicken is simple, too. And I have personally found it no problem at all to switch to low-fat milk and yogurt and reduced-fat cheese and sour cream. But not cracking as many eggs? Actually the egg substitutes today have come a long way and I generally use half real eggs and half egg substitute when I'm cooking at home. Muffins, cakes, quiches, even omelets still turn out terrific.

Big or little results

Keep in mind some people show big changes in their serum cholesterol after dietary cholesterol and saturated fat have been increased or decreased, while others show little changes. Blame or thank your genetics. Some people are more sensitive to the cholesterol-raising effects of foods high in saturated fat and cholesterol.

Step #5: Calories do count

According to a survey by the National Center for Health Statistics, fat in our diet has actually decreased from 36 percent of calories (in 1978) to 34 percent (in 1990). But here's the kicker—Americans were also found to be consuming 231 more calories per person per day. Some researchers argue that Americans are actually eating more calories due to all the fat-free and light products on the market. How can this be? First of all, many of these fat-free products have just as many calories (sometimes more) as the regular versions. And I don't know if you've noticed, but people often end up eating more of these fat-free products compared to regular versions.

Why do some people need to eat so much of these products? Could it be, perhaps, that these foods are less satisfying and so we eat more in hopes of becoming more satisfied? Just a thought. Perhaps we also tend to eat more because we think they can do no harm, no matter what the quantity. Don't get me wrong, I'm a fan of quite a few of the better-tasting reduced fat products, but remember, the benefits of eating lower fat and calorie products are quickly lost with larger serving sizes.

Mind over matter

How does thinking we are eating something very low-fat or fat-free affect our overall intake? In one study, women ate more at lunch when they ate a yogurt labeled "low-fat" than they did after eating the high-fat yogurt—even though the yogurts contained the same number of calories. Perhaps this has something to do with women paying less attention to their actual hunger and more attention to controlling their intake. As someone with diabetes, you are encouraged to calculate grams of carbohydrates (at least) throughout the day. But there is a difference between controlling your intake and counting your intake.

You still need to listen to your hunger cues. If you are hungry, you should eat. When you are no longer hungry, but comfortable, you should stop eating. In terms of counting, though, it is helpful if you are counting what you eat so that you can look back on your after-meal blood sugars and get an idea of how your body handled that particular amount and combination of foods for next time.

Step #6: Eat more fruits and vegetables

Starting your meals/snacks with fruits and vegetables is a trick I've learned with my family. If you start your meal by enjoying fruits and vegetables, you'll be sure to get some and they will help fill you up so you won't be as likely to overeat the meat or entrée. Eating at a pizza parlor is a perfect example. While you are waiting for your pizza, relax and enjoy a nice green salad with tomato, kidney beans, and other vegetables (making sure to keep regular dressings to about a tablespoon). You'll find that you won't eat as much pizza. However, if you eat the salad at the same time you eat your pizza, you are less likely not to eat salad and vegetables.

There are many health reasons to eat more fruits and vegetables (fiber, vitamins and minerals, antioxidants, phytochemicals, and most are naturally low in fat, sugar and sodium). The sad truth is, we already know this. We just don't get around to eating enough fruits and vegetables most days. Most people say it is because they aren't as convenient as snack foods and fast food. Others say they simply aren't in the habit. Well, whatever your reason, the time to change this is now.

Making fruits and vegetables more habit-forming

I think we would all eat better if we just had a personal fruit and vegetable assistant to help us. We need someone to remember to buy the fruits and vegetables, someone to take the time to turn them into beautiful fruit salads or green salads, snack trays, and garnishes or tasty side dishes to our entrées. All this takes time, talent, and love. Here are some ways to make fruits and vegetables a little more convenient:

- Pack your bookbag or locker with your favorite dried fruits; they will keep for weeks.

- Buy baby carrots and celery sticks and put them out before dinner with a quick dip (mix some light or fat-free sour cream with Hidden Valley Ranch dressing powder or onion dip powder to taste).

- Take time Sunday or at the beginning or end of the school week to make a large spinach salad or vegetable-fortified lettuce salad, and just store it (without dressing) in an airtight container. You can have crisp, wonderful salad as a snack or with your lunch or dinner for the next few days.

- Every few days make a point of going to your supermarket and picking out the best tasting and freshest fruits in season. But don't just buy it. Remember you have it and put it out as a snack. Add a few slices or wedges of fruit to each lunch or dinner plate.

- With a few chops of a knife, you can turn a few pieces of fruit into a beautiful fruit salad. Drizzle lemon, pineapple or orange juice over the top and toss to coat the fruit with it (the vitamin C helps prevent browning).

- Buy your favorite fruits in the winter—just buy them frozen or canned in juice or light syrup.

- Stock your refrigerator at work and home with your favorite fruit juices (make sure they are 100-percent juice). You can often buy them in individual servings so you can grab them as you are running out the door.

- Make a point to include a vegetable with your lunch.

- Make sure to enjoy vegetables when you eat out at a restaurant or deli.

For a list of fruits and vegetables rich in soluble fiber, refer back to Step #1 on page 76.

Step #7: Avoid eating large meals

Eating more often, but smaller amounts at a time, is a good idea for every single American but can be particularly helpful for people with type II diabetes.

What small meals do for blood sugar levels

Small meals, spaced throughout the day (about every 2 1/2 to 3 hours,) translate into more stable blood sugars throughout the day. Smaller meals generally result in smaller blood glucose responses, requiring less insulin and improving blood glucose control in people with type II diabetes.

It makes sense that the bigger the meal, the larger the number of calories eaten from carbohydrates, fat, and protein, and the higher the blood levels of those nutrients will be after the "large" meal. Large meals also zap you of your after-meal energy. If you've had a large meal, a nap is usually not far behind. But if you eat smaller meals you will feel more energetic throughout your day. (Smaller, lower fat meals don't stay in the stomach long, they move quickly to the intestines.) If you feel "light" on your feet, you will be more likely to be physically active too. The more physically active, the more calories you will burn going about your day. And don't forget that exercise and activity acts like insulin in the body too.

Other benefits of small meals

If you don't want to eat this way to help your diabetes, then do it for these other great reasons:

- Your brain and body require a constant supply of energy in the blood. Eating smaller, more frequent meals is more likely to keep you blood sugar (and energy) stable—preventing low blood sugar levels (which can trigger headaches, irritability, food cravings, or overeating in susceptible people).

- Eating smaller, more frequent meals is great for appetite control. The more stable blood sugars keep us from getting overly hungry, which can lead to overeating or making high-sugar or high-fat food choices.

- One study observed that obesity was less common in people who ate more frequent meals. People who eat smaller, more frequent meals are less likely to overeat at any meal. Larger meals flood your bloodstream with a load of fat, protein, and carbohydrate calories, and your body has to get rid of any extra calories. What does this have to do with being overweight? All extra calories can be converted to body fat for energy storage.

- This is still being investigated, but it is possible that this eating style may help lower serum cholesterol. It stands to reason that by avoiding large meals you also prevent quick rises of serum triglycerides that typically follow large, particularly fatty meals

- Burn more calories digesting, absorbing, and metabolizing your food just by eating more often. The body burns calories when it digests and absorbs the food we eat. And every time we eat, the digestion process goes into gear. If we eat six small meals instead of two large ones, we start the digestive process three times more often every single day—burning more calories. This metabolism-inspired increase in calories burned can burn around 5 to10 percent of the total calories we eat in a day.

- It's physically more comfortable to eat smaller meals. You aren't weighed down by a large meal in your stomach.

F.Y.I. ## How soon after a meal does your blood glucose peak?

Depending on the exact composition and size of your meal, your blood glucose (blood sugar) begins to rise 30 to 60 minutes after eating and peaks about 1 1/2 to 2 hours after the meal.

How frequent should the "smaller" meals be?

Experts have not yet determined the ideal eating pattern for people with diabetes, but so far it seems that the closer together the meals are, the better the results. The longer the gap between a previous meal or snack and dinner, for example, the larger the dinner typically ends up being.

If you eat a small breakfast, have a midmorning snack, a light lunch, then an afternoon snack, and a light dinner and maybe a nighttime snack—it adds up to six small meals for the day. The best advice I can give you, until researchers know more, is to space your meals according to your individual schedule, when you tend to get hungry, and your blood glucose goals.

Fight the urge to eat at night

We burn 70 percent of our calories as fuel during the day, but when do many Americans eat the majority of their calories? During the evening hours. If we've eaten small meals throughout the day, eating when we were hungry and stopping when we were "comfortable," it should be easier to avoid eating large dinners and evening desserts and snacks. Try to keep in mind that what you eat in the evening will be hitting your bloodstream pretty much around the time you are getting in your jammies. It isn't as though you are eating to fuel a marathon or anything.

When a bedtime snack is in order

If you eat an early dinner, you may need to eat a small bedtime snack. Choose something you tolerate well, like an apple or small bowl of oatmeal. I know it's hard to believe, but this helps reduce early morning blood glucose levels for many people.

Easier said than done

Our whole society is based on three meals a day—with dinner typically being the largest meal of the day. This is a hard habit to break. If you eat out often, it becomes particularly difficult not to eat a large meal. Restaurants tend to serve large meals—that's all there is to it. It requires extra diligence at restaurants to eat only half your meal and save the rest for later. If you are having spaghetti, you could eat the salad and half your entrée, then have the garlic bread and the rest of your spaghetti later or the next day. I'm not saying it isn't going to be difficult—but it can be done.

If you are on insulin or other medications . . .

Your meals and medications need to fit together well. For example, meals need to be spaced according to the type of insulin you are taking and its period of peak action. It is important that you discuss your new eating schedule (eating smaller more frequent meals) with your dietitian or certified diabetes educator first, because he or she can help modify your medications accordingly.

Step #8: Improving your diet with supplements

When you walk into a vitamin supplement store, you're a sitting duck. Remember, the business of selling supplements is a big and lucrative one. The more pills they can talk you into, the thicker their wallets. However, the supplements I'm talking about shouldn't run you very much at all. In fact you can buy them at your local drugstore or supermarket.

Start with a good multivitamin plus minerals

One of the best things you can do for yourself, in the way of supplements, is to just take a good multivitamin with minerals.

Taking a multivitamin with minerals is like having nutrition insurance. We feel better knowing that if we aren't getting enough in our food, at least we are getting some from our multivitamin. Multivitamins have come a long way and many are very balanced and complete and even include recommended amounts of up-and-coming minerals like chromium, selenium, and boron. A 2-month supply will cost you about $3 a month.

Many of the vitamins and minerals you will find in your top-notch multivitamin with minerals may actually help your diabetes:

Chromium. This mineral might make cells more receptive to insulin. Some experts say it does decrease HbA1c levels (200 mcg several times a day) and some say it doesn't. More studies are needed because of chromium's unproven benefits and unknown risks. You can get about 65–120 mcg of chromium in your multivitamin.

Magnesium. A deficiency of this mineral may contribute to hypertension. If a person's diet is deficient it may also make cells more resistant to insulin. Your multivitamin contains about 100 mg (25 percent of the RDA).

Antioxidants. Some researchers think people with diabetes use up their antioxidant stores more quickly, increasing their requirements (sort of like smokers do). They think this happens with diabetes because the disease creates more free radicals, which use up the vitamins. With high levels of glucose in the blood, it is thought that some of the glucose molecules bind onto proteins and lipids (called glycosylation), making them more susceptible to oxidation. This oxidation process generates more free radicals.

Vitamin C. Some researchers have found that 250 to 500 milligrams of vitamin C reduce glycosylation. Most multivitamins contain at least 60 milligrams.

Vitamin E. This antioxidant has been associated with many heart disease prevention benefits at the level of 200 to 400 IU per day, but some researchers say that supplementation may also improve blood sugars. Most multivitamins contain 30 to 45 IU.

Selenium is an important antioxidant. Some multivitamins contain about 20 mcg per pill.

Folic acid acts like an antioxidant in the body. It is known (along with the B vitamins) for assisting in the lowering of elevated homocysteine levels in the body. (High levels of homocysteine are associated with increased risk of heart disease.) Two groups of people are known to have problems with elevated homocysteine levels: people with a rare genetic problem that causes early heart attacks, and people with diabetes. More needs to be known about the benefits of folic acid for people with diabetes, but one researcher reported that folic acid may help with vascular disease in people with type II diabetes. Your basic multivitamin contains 400 mcg.

Reading the label

When you are shopping for your multivitamin with minerals, ask yourself these questions:

Does it contain the known antioxidants?

Look for vitamin A (some of which is beta carotene), vitamin E, vitamin C, and selenium.

Does it contain chromium?

Even though we don't yet have a daily recommended amount for the mineral chromium, it is important your supplement have at least the minimum suggested by the Recommended Daily Allowance committee—50 micrograms.

Does it contain 100 percent of the daily value for most of the vitamins and minerals and, if it doesn't, does it have a good reason to include more or less?

There are some exceptions. Biotin will only be at 10 percent daily value because it is very expensive, and you won't find calcium or magnesium in amounts much greater than 25 percent daily value because they add so much bulk. (If they did include 100 percent of the daily value, they would look more like horse pills.)

How much iron does it contain?

You will mostly likely need multivitamins with 100 percent daily value of iron.

How much of the "bone building" micronutrients— calcium, magnesium, and vitamin D—does it contain? Does it include enough vitamin D?

As we age, we lose the ability to make vitamin D through our skin. The daily recommended intake (DRI) for vitamin D is 200 IU for males and females ages nine to eighteen. Most multivitamins contain 400 IU.

The following is a list of the vitamin/mineral content of a few widely available supplements. All three score pretty well on the previous questions. See which one meets your own personal needs best.

Supplementing vitamin E

Many researchers are recommending about 400 IU of vitamin E for potential immune and heart disease prevention benefits. Two of the supplements in the following chart only contain 30 to 60 IU. In the best of nutritional circumstances, you can only hope to take in about 30 IU from food, leaving a gap of over 300 IU. You can find mixed tocopherol and vitamin E supplements at most grocery or drugstores at about $2 per one-month supply.

Warning: The beneficial anti-clotting effect of vitamin E could pose a danger for people on blood-thinning medications (anticoagulants). If you are on any medications affecting blood clotting, you probably shouldn't take vitamin E supplements, but check with your doctor. When you are taking an aspirin a day (to help keep the cardiologist away), which also has an anticoagulant effect, you aren't usually taking enough of it to make vitamin E a problem. But if you are taking high doses of a pain reliever for chronic pain, talk to your doctor first about vitamin E supplements.

Multivitamin/Mineral Supplements for Teens			
Nutrient	**GNC Teens Mega Teen Multivitamin**	**Rainbow Light Active Health Teen Multivitamin**	**Pediatrician's Choice Teens Multivitamin**
Vitamin A	5000 IU	10,000 IU	5000 IU
Vitamin C	75 mg	400 mg	120 mg
Vitamin D	400 IU	100 IU	400 IU
Vitamin E	30 IU	200 IU	60 IU
B-6	6 mg (300%)	20 mg	6 mg
B-12	18 mcg (300%)	60 mcg	18 mcg
Folic Acid	400 mcg	400 mcg	400 mcg
Calcium	200 mg	200 mg	39 mg
Magnesium	50 mg (13%)	200 mg (50%)	40 mg (10%)
Zinc	15 mg	15 mg	15 mg
Selenium	70 mcg	200 mcg	70 mcg
Chrominum	120 mcg	100 mcg	120 mcg
Niacin	20 mcg	100 mcg	40 mcg
Iron	18 mg	N/A	18 mg

One powerful antioxidant

Alphalipoic acid is being billed by several researchers as a very strong antioxidant that helps fight insulin resistance and neuropathy. That's quite a tall order. Early studies are showing that it is indeed useful for people with diabetic neuropathy (nerve damage). One study in lean and obese people with type II diabetes found lower fasting blood sugars in both groups when 600 milligrams were taken twice a day. There were more drastic changes, however, in the lean group. There aren't many studies on alphalipoic acid yet, but so far, the results seem consistent. If you are interested in this antioxidant supplement, you absolutely need to work closely with your diabetes educator, because it could potentially lower blood sugars and you need to be closely monitored.

Try flaxseed

If you haven't heard of flaxseed yet, trust me you will. I predict flaxseed will be to the 21st century what wheat germ was to the 60s. It is just now being studied in humans, mostly for its blood lipid lowering benefits and tumor-reducing properties with some types of cancer. (It seems to be so effective in reducing estrogen and lowering breast cancer risk that it is now being tested clinically to shrink breast cancer tumors before surgery on women just diagnosed with breast cancer.) We will know much more about flaxseed's health benefits in 10 more years. But that is then and this is now.

Flaxseed has actually been around and used by humans as food and medicine for hundreds of years. Twelve centuries ago Charlemagne decreed that all loyal Romans should eat it to guard their health. It is looking like these were very wise words indeed, from a civilization that didn't have million-dollar, double-blind studies to test their theories.

At this point what they had were personal observations. Flaxseed was cataloged by physician Nicholas Culpeper, in the 1600s in his book *Complete Herbal*—"Flaxseed is of great use against inflammations, tumors, and imposthumes, and is frequently put into fomentations and cataplasms" (abscesses, compresses, and poultices).

What is it about the flaxseed that might be responsible for all this? We know that flaxseed is an extraordinary source of phytoestrogens—lignans—containing 75 to 800 times as much as other plant sources. Lignans are also considered to act as antioxidants, protecting healthy cells from chance meetings with free radicals in the body.

Flaxseed is also packed with the plant form of omega-3 fatty acids, alpha-linolenic acid. In fact, about half of the oil in flaxseed is alpha-linolenic acid. It is possible the fish form of omega-3s is more powerful in the body, but it looks like the plant form offers the benefits too. The omega-3s in flaxseed help prevent blood clots that might lead to heart attacks, according to University of Toronto nutrition researcher Stephen Cunnane, Ph.D. The omega-3s do this by helping make platelets (a component in the blood) less likely to stick together, causing a chain reaction that leads to a blood clot.

Flaxseed is, at the very least, a good source of soluble fiber, which may help lower cholesterol and blood sugar levels. When women in Cunnane's study added about two tablespoons of ground flax to their daily diet for four weeks, their total cholesterol fell 9 percent and their LDL ("bad" cholesterol) dropped 18 percent (while HDL "good" cholesterol stayed the same). These same results were also found in a different study conducted by researchers in the United States.

Flaxseed may also make our arteries more flexible—something that would potentially lead to a decrease risk of heart attack and stroke—after supplementing your diet with it for just one month. You've heard of "hardening of the arteries"—a stiffening of blood vessel walls caused by high blood pressure, diabetes, and/or atherosclerosis (a type of plaquing in the arteries). Well, flaxseed may help make the arteries less "hard." More research needs to be done on this though, but so far so good.

Once you grind the seeds (and you'll want to because the body enzymes can get to the beneficial chemicals better this way), it is perishable and can be kept in the freezer in a airtight container for up to two months. If you opt for flaxseed oil, remember that it doesn't contain the beneficial lignans and fiber because they are both removed in the process of making the oil. Because we want all the benefits from flaxseed, I recommend buying whole (to be ground at home) or ground flaxseeds, not flaxseed oil.

You will find the seeds (often in bulk bins) in health food stores. If you buy them whole, you'll need to store them in the refrigerator and grind them up yourself, in a spice or coffee bean grinder—perhaps a few day's supply at a time. (I recommend having a designated flax grinder for this.) Store the ground seeds in a resealable bag, in the refrigerator, and scoop out two to three teaspoons a day, which you can then proceed to stir into some juice, sprinkle over some hot or cold cereal, or whip up in a breakfast smoothie. You can also bake a daily ration (or half a ration) of flaxseed into each serving of bread or muffin.

You might even be able to find a product called "Fortified Flax," which is a preground flaxseed (that looks like cornmeal). It is fortified with nutrients such as vitamin C and E, to stabilize it against oxidation, which keeps it from going rancid. Once a package of preground

F.Y.I. How much flax is enough?

Flax researchers are considering 1-2 tablespoons a day of ground flaxseed to be "safe and effective."

If flaxseed had a nutrition information label it might look something like this:

1 tablespoon:
Calories: 40
Protein: 1.6 g
Carbohydrates: 2.8 g
Total fat: 2.8 g
Omega-3 fatty acids: 1.5 g
Monounsaturated fat: .6 g
Saturated fat: .3 g
Fiber: 2.3 g (1/3 of which is soluble, the rest is insoluble)
Cholesterol: 0 mg
Folic acid: 15 percent daily value
Magnesium: 12.5 percent daily value
Phosphorus: 6 percent daily value
Vitamin B6: 6 percent daily value
Vitamin E: 6 percent daily value
Total lignans (phytoestrogens): 6,600 mcg

Warning: Some people are highly allergic to flax, so start with 1/4 teaspoon a day and increase the amount gradually if you don't have a reaction. Another reason you want to start off slowly is that flaxseed, which is high in fiber, can cause gassiness and bloating if you aren't used to it.

flaxseed is opened, keep it refrigerated, and whatever you don't use in six months, throw away.

But how does it taste? You won't mind the sprinkle or two. Flaxseed has a nice nutty taste to it. For the latest scientific information, practical tips, and lots of flax recipes, check out my new cookbook, *The Flax Cookbook* (Marlowe & Co. 2003)!

Step #9: Monitor your blood sugars

Keeping your blood glucose as near to normal as possible protects your body from diabetic complications further down the line. Measuring your blood sugar levels on a fairly regular basis, then, is a necessary step toward tightly controlling your blood sugar. Measuring your blood sugars will tell you whether you are meeting your treatment goals and whether the agreed-upon treatments (diet, exercise, or pharmacological) are working.

You are hopefully working with a dietitian or diabetes educator who is helping you personalize your eating plan. Logging in your food, blood sugars, medications and exercise per day shows your dietitian or diabetes educator how your blood sugar is being affected from day to day. They can then work with you on fine-tuning your diabetes care plan (by adjusting medications, changing your desired amount of carbohydrate grams, and encouraging activity at certain times).

About 1 1/2 hours after eating you will know whether your blood sugar is within normal limits, high, or low. This is your greatest tool! Use it. Each of us reacts a little differently to each food, combination of foods, and amount of those foods. The only way you can learn your own personal reaction to a particular meal is to test your blood sugar 1 1/2 hours later. Once you begin testing and recording your blood sugar levels, you can look back to your records for clues to why your readings are what they are. Look for clues in three areas:

1. Food and diet. (What foods and how much?)
2. A change in your exercise or activity schedule. (Did you exercise at your usual time for the usual length?)
3. Medication. (Did you take the proper amount of medication at the proper time?)

Make sure someone on your healthcare team clearly demonstrates how to measure your glucose and how to record it so it can be referred to easily at follow-up visits.

Step #10: Make exercise fun, and do it every day!

When you exercise regularly, you just plain feel better. You burn more calories and you increase your muscle mass, which increases your metabolic rate. And that's just the beginning. Exercising will help decrease blood sugar levels and possibly the dose of insulin you need to take (if you take insulin). It will decrease blood cholesterol levels and bone loss while improving your circulation, heart function, and your ability to deal with stress. Obviously exercise has huge health pay offs.

Make exercise a priority, please! Start making it a habit to exercise. Get a schedule going, like walking with a friend on Tuesdays and Thursdays, and going to an exercise class on Mondays and Wednesdays.

Recommendations for exercise

If you are currently sedentary and want to start exercising just enough to improve your risk factors for chronic diseases, exercise:

Frequency: 2 to 3 times a week.
Intensity: 40 percent maximum heart rate.
Duration: 15-30 minutes.

If you want to be physically fit, exercise:
Frequency: 4 times a week.
Intensity: 70-90 percent maximum heart rate.
Duration: 15-30 minutes.

If you want specifically to lose weight, exercise:
Frequency: 5 times a week.
Intensity: 45-60 percent maximum heart rate.
Duration: 45-60 minutes.

Resistance training recommendations

Perform one set of 8 to 12 repetitions of 8 to 10 exercises that condition the major muscle groups, at least two days a week, minimum.

4 reasons why many people don't exercise

1. It isn't fun!

It isn't exercise, per se, that isn't fun; it's the type of exercise that you have been doing (or not doing) that you are not finding fun. Think about all the possible types of exercise and write down which ones you might find the most fun. Also think about what types of exercise you don't like—and try to put your finger on why you might not be finding it fun. This will give you some clues about what your "fun" exercise options might require.

If you dislike the types of exercise that you do alone, then perhaps you would like exercise that is done as group or team. If you don't think exercising at home is fun, then you should think about exercise that you can do somewhere close to your home—pool aerobics, walking with a buddy, country western dance lessons, and so on.

2. There's just no time!

We make time for the things we really want to do, don't we? And we make time for the things we really have to do too. If exercising makes us feel better (and we make it fun), then hopefully it will become something we really want to do. If exercising helps us control our blood sugar and body weight (and it does!) then it is also something we really have to do—for our health.

Keep in mind that fitting even 10 minutes of exercise here and there, during our day, can help your body manage diabetes. Walking after a meal or snack (or during a time when your blood sugar tends to be too high) can be particularly helpful for diabetics. The exercise acts like insulin in the body, helping move and use the blood sugar in your bloodstream. This doesn't have to be jogging or swimming right after a meal, it could be a quick 10 minute jaunt around your school building after lunch, taking the stairs, walking the dog after dinner, and such.

Instead of "just whistle while you work . . ." how about "just walk while you work." Think about school work, conversations, or informal meetings that you can conduct on foot. Take your brainstorming session to the streets. You'd be surprised what some fresh air will do for your creativity. If you are visiting with a neighbor or a friend pops in for a visit, suggest that you take a walk around your neighborhood while you catch up.

3. It's boring!

Some people get bored more easily than others do. I know—I'm one of them. You may be someone who needs to plan variety into your exercise program. You might want to join a class or league (dance, jazzercise, water aerobics, swimming, golf, basketball, or tennis) that meets two or three days a week, then fill in the other days with walks, weight training, rowing machine, stationary bicycling, stair climbing, etc. Take lessons for a sport you actually find interesting.

For many of us, exercising at home on a machine is most convenient. There is no commute time involved, it doesn't matter if it rains, and once you pay for the machine, you exercise for free. If you work out for 30 minutes, then it takes exactly 30 minutes out of your day. We productive types love this! The problem is, this can get a little boring. You ride your bike and row your stationary boat—but you don't actually go anywhere. There's nothing but the wall in front of you to look at. Or is there?

I ride my stationary bike (some of you might find an incumbent bike more comfortable) while I watch a television movie or program that I'm dying to see. I even fast forward through the commercials if I'm watching a tape. The television keeps my interest while my body is doing the work. If I'm watching something really interesting, the 30 minutes seems to fly by. My husband exercises on his rowing machine while listening to his favorite radio station (something he doesn't get to do very often). You may want to listen to some of your favorite CDs or maybe even an audio book.

4. It's raining, it's pouring!

Having several types of exercise options available to you not only adds variety (and minimizes boredom), it gives you an automatic "bad weather" plan. If you have home exercise equipment, use them when the weather is cold or wet. If you have signed up for exercise classes or sports leagues, they are usually indoors, so you know you will at least get some exercise on those days each week.

If you like to walk and you have a walking buddy depending on you, you could very well decide to walk rain or shine. As long as it isn't raining too hard, my walking buddy and I just put our hooded ski jackets on and brave the drops. I find it invigorating! And the warm shower afterwards is truly therapeutic.

Chapter 5

The 26 Recipes You Can't Live Without

This chapter is designed to give you just a sampling of possible recipes to start you on the road to more healthful cooking. Some of the recipes are wholesome and from scratch while others make use of the countless convenient products now available. Hopefully you will find a handful that suit you perfectly. I have a couple of new cookbooks that might also come in handy: *The Flax Cookbook* (Marlowe & Co., 2002) and *The Recipe Doctor* (Adams Media, 2000), and *Lighten Up!* (Fireside, 1997).

Most of us cook the same recipes over and over again, so I wanted to give you some recipe guidelines to lighten up your own favorites!

Smart substitutions

Healthy food isn't going to do anyone any good if no one is eating it. That's been my motto for the 15 years or so that I've been lightening recipes. In other words, even if it's light, it's gotta taste great.

Lightening recipes comes down to basically two things: (1.) trimming extra fat and fat-containing ingredients and (2.) trimming extra sugar and sugar-containing ingredients. The keys to successful lightening are:

- Find the ideal fat and sugar threshold for the recipe. How much can you cut calories, fat, and sugar without compromising flavor and texture? See the following table for more help on this.

- Use the fat substitute that works best in that recipe. See the table for more help on this also.

- Review the functions of each fatty or sweet ingredient before you make changes to your recipe. When fat or sugar serves an irreplaceable function, you'll probably need to keep some of it in, but you can usually cut fat in half and sugar by one-fourth.

- Substitute reduced-fat and reduced-sugar ingredients and products when appropriate. For example, use reduced-fat sharp cheddar cheese instead of regular, use a good tasting fat-free or light sour cream instead of regular, or use fat-free half-and half. You can also use reduced-calorie pancake syrup, unsweetened frozen fruit, etc., instead of regular.

- When possible, change to a cooking method that eliminates the need for cooking fat (broiling, roasting, poaching, steaming). But when it is necessary to maintain the character of the food, do use a cooking method that involves fat—just use less of it (oven frying, sautéing or pan frying in less fat, or browning).

Ideal fat thresholds and substitutions

Based on two decades of experimentation with the best ways to lighten recipes, I've discovered there are ideal fat thresholds that you must keep for flavor. If you cut back the fat in a particular recipe, you'll need a "fat replacement" (an extra ingredient you can add to help replace the fat you have taken out).

Example #1

If you are making brownies and you cut the butter back from 8 tablespoons to 3, you can add 5 tablespoons fat free sour cream to the batter to make up the difference.

Example #2

If you are making a spice cake using a cake mix, don't add the 1/2 cup of oil the recipe requires; instead add 1/2 cup of unsweetened applesauce (or some other fat replacement) instead.

Recipe	Fat threshold	Fat replacements
Biscuits/Scones	4 Tbs. shortening for every 2 cups flour.	Fat-free cream cheese, nonfat or light sour cream, flavored yogurt.
Cake mixes	No additional fat is needed because most mixes already contain fat in the mix.	Instead of adding the oil called for on the box, add apple-sauce, fruit juice, flavored yogurt, or nonfat sour cream, depending on the cake.
Brownies	2 1/2 Tbs. canola oil or butter per 4 oz. unsweetened chocolate and about 14 Tbs. flour.	Fat-free sour cream works well, along with espresso or strong coffee.
Homemade cakes and coffee cakes	1/4 to 1/3 cup fat ingredient per cake.	Light sour cream for chocolate cakes; fruit purees and juices work well with carrot, apple, and spice cakes.

(cont'd)

Recipe	Fat threshold	Fat replacements
Cheese sauce	No butter is needed, so omit the butter if it is called for—the cheese is the vital fatty ingredient; use a reduced-fat cheddar.	Make your thickening paste by mixing the flour with a little bit of milk, then whisk in the remaining milk called for in the recipe.
Cookies	Generally you can only cut the fat by half. If the original recipe calls for 1 cup of butter, for example, try cutting it to 1/2 cup.	Fat-free cream cheese for rich cookies; some fruit purees may work in fruit/drop cookies.
Marinades	1 Tbs. oil per cup of marinade (or none at all).	Fruit juices help to balance the sharpness of the more acid ingredients in a marinade, such as vinegar or tomato juice.
Muffins and nut bread	2 Tbs. oil for a 12-muffin recipe.	Fat-free sour cream, low-fat flavored yogurts, fruit juice, and fruit purees.
Vinaigrette dressings	1 to 2 Tbs. olive oil per 1/2 cup dressing.	Fruit juice, fruit purees (raspberry and pear work well).
White sauces	1 tsp. butter per serving of sauce.	Add a little more milk; I like to use whole milk or fat-free half-and-half for a rich white sauce.

Here are four more substitution or fat-reduction tips to use when cooking various dishes:

- In mostly egg dishes, you can cut the eggs in half and replace the lost eggs with Egg Beaters egg substitute (1/4 cup substitute per egg).

- Many recipes call for using much more oil or butter in pan frying or sautéing than is really necessary. Using a teaspoon of olive or canola oil, at the most, usually does the trick.

- Canola or olive oil cooking sprays help lubricate bakeware, cookware, and food surfaces with a minimal amount of fat.

- If you can switch to canola or olive oil instead of using fat or shortening in a recipe, do it! These oils contain better fats (omega-3s) than the saturated fats in shortening, butter, and stick margarines.

Stuff the turkey, not yourself

The holidays are the no-holds-barred times of year when we break any food rules we may have during the year. We are celebrating the season and with all the festivities, overindulgence is sure to follow—along with weight gain. Stuffing ourselves with food we don't eat but once a year, eating lots of rich, fatty food, and eating into the night . . . does this sound familiar?

Think about how we eat during the holday seasons. We do exactly the opposite of our healthy eating plan:

- We indulge in high-fat, high-calorie foods.

- We literally "feast" at our holiday feasts—eating large amounts of food at one sitting.

- We often eat these extra-large meals in the evening, just a few hours before we turn in for the night.

- We tend to celebrate by drinking festive beverages, which usually come with a high calorie content.
- We dine out and at other people's homes more than usual during the holiday seasons. In both situations the cooks are usually not concerned with healthy and lower calorie cooking.

So what can you do?

Easy ways to lighten up the holidays

Tip #1: Stop eating around 7 p.m.

This will help cut down on needless "extras" (extra desserts, second helpings, and extra calories).

Tip #2: Ask for a sliver.

If there is a wonderful food, dessert, or appetizer that you really want, try a "sliver" portion and eat it slowly so you really enjoy it. You don't need a large portion of something to satisfy your curiosity.

Tip #3: Beware of beverages.

You would be amazed how quickly calories from drinks and beverages can add up. Drinks with calories are usually either high in sugar or fat. With all the yummy food around, do you really want to spend a big portion of your calorie budget on drinks? Choose noncalorie beverages instead. Seltzer water with a twist of lemon or lime tastes and looks great but contributes zero calories. There are also other no- or low-calorie drink options besides water: unsweetened or artificially sweeetened iced tea, hot tea, decaffeinated coffee (or caffeinated coffee, if you prefer), and of course, diet soft drinks.

Tip #4: Relax during the holidays as much as possible.

Emotional stress and anxiety can aggravate bad eating habits such as compulsive overeating or undereating.

Tip #5: Whatever you do, keep exercising!

Staying on track with your exercise program is particularly important during the holidays. This will help reduce stress and keep your metabolic rate (the amount of calories you burn just maintaining your body) high.

Tip #6: Keep portions to a minimum.

As hard and as impossible as this sounds, try not to eat those "eat till you explode" large meals. Passing up "seconds" will usually do the trick. I know everything tastes so good, so bring some leftovers home and enjoy the whole dinner again—tommorrow.

Tip #7: Make better choices.

When confronted with the typical holiday nibbles, know which ones are more likely to fit into your healthy eating plan (dishes that are lower in fat, higher in fiber, and higher in important nutrients).

Tip #8: B.Y.O.D.

Offer to bring your own dish to the party or holiday meal that you know would be a healthier choice. You can bring lower fat/lower calorie renditions of favorite holiday foods (See the recipes on pages 124–131).

Tip #9: Try ingredient substitutions.

It's amazing what a difference (in calories and fat grams) a few ingredient substitutions can make. Here are a few examples:

- Use light cream cheese (instead of regular) in your holiday dips, spreads, and cheesecakes to cut out about 16 grams of fat per cup of cream cheese.

- Use a great tasting fat-free sour cream for dips, spreads, and potato dishes to cut out about 320 calories and about 35 grams of fat per cup of sour cream.

- Use reduced-fat cheese in your appetizers and side dishes to cut out 36 grams of fat and 320 calories for every 8 ounces.

- Make your dips, side dishes, and appetizers with a mixture of real mayonnaise and fat-free sour cream. (For every cup of mayo, blend 1/4 cup mayo with 3/4 cup fat-free sour cream.) This mixture will cut out more than 1,000 calories and 132 grams of fat per cup of mayonnaise.

By simply making a few recipe adjustments, you can transform many of your favorite holiday dishes into tasty dishes with half the fat and fewer calories. Here are some holiday recipes to get you started:

Holiday goodies

 ## Potato Latkes

The original recipe called for 3 eggs and 1/2 cup peanut oil. I used 1 egg, 6 tablespoons egg substitute, and 2 to 3 teaspoons canola oil. I also decreased the salt from 1 1/2 teaspoons to 1 teaspoon (but you can cut it down further or leave it out if you are cooking for someone on a low sodium diet). These were delicious and really easy to make!

Makes 10 latkes.

- 2 cups russet potatoes, peeled, shredded, and firmly packed (about 1 pound)
- 1/4 cup onion, grated or finely chopped
- 1 large egg
- 1 Tbs. egg substitute
- 2 to 3 Tbs. low-sodium matzo meal (a little less than 1 matzo), processed into fine crumbs
- 1 tsp. salt
- 2 to 3 tsp. canola oil

1. Place the potatoes in a cheesecloth or double thickness of paper towels and wring to extract as much water out of the potatoes as possible.

2. In medium bowl, stir the potatoes, onion, egg, egg substitute, matzo meal, and salt.

3. In a large heavy-bottomed non-stick skillet, over medium-high heat, heat the oil. Make sure the oil is spread evenly over the bottom of the skillet. Place 1/4 cup (level measure) of potato mixture into the hot oil, pressing down on them to form 1/4- to 1/2-inch thick patties. Spray tops with canola cooking spray. Brown on one side for about 3 minutes. Turn over and brown the other side (about 3 minutes).

4. Serve these hot with applesauce, fat-free or light sour cream, and chopped green onions.

Per latke (if 2 tsp. of canola used): 71 calories, 3 g protein, 12 g carbohydrate, 1.5 g fat (.2 g saturated fat, .7 g monounsaturated fat, .4 g polyunsaturated fat), 21 mg cholesterol, 1 g fiber, 237 mg sodium. Calories from fat: 19 percent.

Original recipe: 121 calories, 7 grams fat, and 63 mg cholesterol per latke.

Hash Brown Casserole

This is a favorite holiday side dish in many homes across the country. In this light version, we used Healthy Request cream of celery soup, reduced-fat sharp cheddar cheese (and less of it), and fat-free sour cream. It's bubbly and golden brown on top and totally irresistible!

Makes 12 servings.

- 1 can (10 3/4 ounces) Healthy Request cream of celery soup, condensed
- 2 cups (8 ounces) reduced-fat sharp cheddar cheese, grated

- 1 cup fat-free or light sour cream
- 1 cup onion, finely chopped
- 1 30-oz. (or 2-lb.) bag of frozen shredded hash brown potatoes, unthawed
- 1 ounce regular or reduced-fat potato chips, crushed into coarse crumbs
1. Preheat oven to 350 degrees. Coat a 13 x 9 x 2-inch baking dish with canola cooking spray.
2. Combine soup, cheese, sour cream, and onion in a large bowl and blend well; fold in the hash browns.
3. Spread mixture into prepared baking dish and bake about 1 hour. Sprinkle top of casserole evenly with potato chip crumbs and bake until golden brown and bubbly (about 5 to 10 minutes).

Per serving: 186 calories, 8 g protein, 24.5 g carbohydrate, 6 g fat (3.3 g saturated fat, .3 g monounsaturated fat, .7 g polyunsaturated fat), 16 mg cholesterol, 2 g fiber, 392 mg sodium. Calories from fat: 29 percent.

Original recipe: 330 calories, 22 grams fat, 11 grams saturated fat, and 41 mg cholesterol per serving.

 ## Green Bean Casserole

I couldn't believe how a few ingredient changes made such a big difference in fat grams. I also doubled the amount of onion and switched to frozen French style green beans instead of canned, which is what the original recipe called for, but you can choose for yourself.

Makes 9 side servings.

- 1 Tbs. butter
- 1 cup fat-free or light sour cream

- 2 Tbs. Wondra quick-mixing flour (regular flour can also be used)
- 1 tsp. salt
- 1 tsp. granulated sugar
- 1/2 cup chopped onion
- 1 16-oz. bag of frozen French style green beans (if you prefer, use 3 14.5-oz. cans, drained)
- 1 cup shredded reduced fat cheddar cheese
- 1/2 cup crumbled reduced-fat Ritz crackers (or similar), about 10 crackers
- Canola cooking spray

1. Preheat oven to 350 degrees. Coat a 9 x 9-inch baking dish with canola cooking spray.
2. In microwave, melt 1 Tbs. of butter in a 2-cup glass measure. Stir in 2 Tbs. of the sour cream and the flour. Add remaining sour cream, salt, and sugar, and stir until well blended.
3. In large bowl, blend the sour cream mixture with the green beans and half the cheddar cheese. Spread mixture into prepared baking dish.
4. Spread remaining cheese over the top of mixture and top that with the cracker crumbs. Spray the cracker topping lightly with canola cooking spray.
5. Bake for 30 to 35 minutes or until the top is golden and sauce is bubbly.

Per serving: 115 calories, 6 g protein, 13.5 g carbohydrate, 4 g fat (2.2 g saturated fat, 1.1 g monounsaturated fat, .1 g polyunsaturated fat), 10 mg cholesterol, 1.5 g fiber, 368 mg sodium. Calories from fat: 31 percent.

Original Recipe: 208 calories, 16.5 grams fat, and 43 milligrams cholesterol per serving.

Best Cornbread Dressing

(From *Chez Moi—Lightening Up Recipes from Famous Restaurants,* Elaine Magee, Cumberland House, 1999.)

This is one of the best darned dressings I've tasted. Even people who don't care for cornbread enjoy this dressing!

Makes 10 servings.

- 8 slices bread, torn or cut into small pieces
- 6 cups cornbread, cooked and crumbled
- 5 chicken-flavored bouillon cubes or 2 Tbs. chicken broth base
- 4 cups boiling water
- 1 large onion, chopped
- 2 stalks celery, chopped
- 1 Tbs. canola oil (olive oil, butter, or margarine can be substituted)
- 1 to 2 tsp. ground sage
- 1 tsp. baking powder
- 2 eggs, beaten
- 1/2 cups egg substitute
- 1/2 tsp. salt (optional)
- 1/4 tsp. pepper (add more to taste)

1. Preheat oven to 350 degrees. Coat a 9 x 13-inch baking dish with canola cooking spray. Set aside.

2. In a large bowl, combine the cornbread crumbs and bread pieces. Dissolve the bouillon cubes in boiling water. Pour the bouillon over the crumb mixture and stir well.

3. In a nonstick skillet or frying pan, saute the onion and celery in butter over medium heat until tender. Add to the crumb mixture.

4. Stir in the remaining ingredients (adjust sage and other seasoning to your taste preference).

5. Spoon into the prepared pan. Bake for about 45 minutes. Serve!

Per serving: 209 calories, 7.5 g protein, 30 grams carbohydrate, 6.5 g fat, 2 g saturated fat, 67 mg cholesterol, 3 g fiber, 890 mg sodium (you can reduce the sodium by using reduced sodium chicken broth powder). Calories from fat: 29 percent.

Original recipe: around 415 calories, 33 grams fat, and 83 milligrams cholesterol per serving.

 ## Light Libby's Pumpkin Pie

(From Elaine Magee's *Lighten Up!*, Fireside, 1997.)

By using egg substitute, evaporated skimmed milk, and a lightened buttermilk pie crust, I've elminated half the fat grams, but saved the rich, spicy taste we all love.

Makes 10 servings.

- 1/2 cup egg substitute
- 1 16-ounce can Libby's solid-pack pumpkin
- 3/4 cup sugar
- 1 tsp. ground cinnamon
- 1/2 tsp. ground ginger
- 1/4 tsp. ground cloves
- 1/2 tsp. salt
- 1 12-ounce can undiluted evaporated skim milk
- 1 1/2 tsp. grated orange zest (optional)
- 1 unbaked 9-inch Light and Flaky Piecrust (page 130)

1. Preheat oven to 425 degrees.

2. In a large bowl, combine the egg substitute, pumpkin, sugar, cinnamon, ginger, cloves, salt, and evaporated milk, and beat just until smooth.

Stir in the orange zest if desired. Pour into the prepared pie crust.

3. Bake for 15 minutes (if using a metal or foil pan, bake on a preheated heavy-duty baking sheet). Reduce the oven temperature to 350 degrees; bake for 40 minutes longer, or until a knife inserted near the center comes out clean. Cool on a wire rack.

Per serving: 171 calories, 6.5 g protein, 21 g carbohydrate, 6.8 g fat, 7.5 mg cholesterol, 1.3 g fiber, 180 mg sodium. Calories from fat: 36 percent.

Original recipe: 232 calories, 53 mg cholesterol, and 14.5 grams of fat per serving.

By replacing some of the shortening with fat-free cream cheese and low-fat buttermilk, I've cut down on the calories and fat without sacrificing taste or texture.

 ## Light and Flaky Buttermilk Pie Crust

- 1 1/3 cups all purpose flour, sifted
- 1/2 tsp. salt
- 5 Tbs. butter-flavor Crisco (butter or canola margarine may also be used)
- 3 Tbs. fat-free cream cheese
- 3 to 4 Tbs. low-fat buttermilk

1. Combine the flour and salt in a medium bowl. With a pastry blender or two knives, cut in the Crisco and cream cheese until uniform; the mixture should resemble coarse meal.

2. Sprinkle with the buttermilk, a tablespoon at a time, and toss with a fork just until the dough comes together. Knead in any dry crumbs.

3. Lay a sheet of waxed paper over a flat surface and lightly flour the waxed paper. Roll the dough

into a circle to fit a 9-inch pie plate. Gently ease the dough into the plate (you make have to use a spatula to lift up the dough). Trim the dough to 1/2-inch beyond the edge of the plate; fold under to make a double thickness of dough around rim and flute with your fingers or crimp with a fork.

Continue with previous recipe for Light Libby's Pumpkin Pie.

Flaxseed recipes

 ### Honey Wheat Bread with Flaxseed

I must have experimented with a dozen different bread machine wheat bread recipes and none were great enough for this book—that is, until I found this one! (For two-pound bread machines.)

Makes 12 slices.

- 1 1/8 cups water
- 2 1/2 cups white bread flour
- 1/2 cup whole wheat flour
- 1 1/2 Tbs. dry milk
- 1 1/2 Tbs. honey
- 1 1/2 tsp. salt
- 2 Tbs. canola oil
- 1/4 cup ground flaxseed
- 3 tsp. active dry yeast (or 2 tsp. fast-rise yeast)

1. Measure your ingredients and one after the other, load them into your bread machine pan. Add them in the order suggested in your machine owner's manual. (Usually you add the liquids first and end with the dry ingredients. Make a well in your flour and add the yeast.)

2. Adjust the setting for "wheat bread" and then press "Start." This recipe can also be made with rapid or delayed time bake cycles.

3. Let the bread cool slightly before removing from the pan. Use a serrated knife to cut into about 12 slices. Enjoy this bread with canola margarine, reduced-fat peanut butter, your favorite preserves, or make your favorite sandwich.

Per serving: 150 calories, 5 g protein, 25 g carbohydrate, 3.8 g fat, .5 g saturated fat, 1 mg cholesterol, 2 g fiber, 280 mg sodium. Calories from fat: 19 percent. .5 grams omega-3 fatty acid per slice (1 g per sandwich).

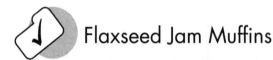 Flaxseed Jam Muffins

Makes 9 regular sized muffins.
- Canola cooking spray
- 1/8 cup nonfat or light sour cream
- 1/8 cup canola oil
- 1/2 cup low-fat milk
- 1/4 cup egg substitute (or 1 egg)
- 2 Tbs. light corn syrup
- 1 tsp. vanilla extract
- 2/3 cup unbleached flour
- 2/3 cup whole wheat flour
- 1/3 cup ground flaxseed
- 1/2 cup granulated sugar
- 2 tsp. baking powder
- 1/2 tsp. salt
- 4 Tbs. jam of your choice

1. Preheat oven to 375 degrees. Coat 9 muffin cups with canola cooking spray.

2. Place sour cream in a glass mixing bowl and warm briefly in the microwave so it will blend easier. Stir in oil and milk, a tablespoon at a time. Stir in egg or egg substitute, corn syrup, and vanilla extract.

3. Blend dry ingredients together (flours, flaxseed, sugar, baking powder, salt) and add all at once to liquid mixture. Stir just enough to moisten.

4. Fill each muffin cup with a level 1/4 cup measure of batter. Spoon about 1 1/2 teaspoons jam in the center of each muffin. Bake about 18 to 20 minutes or until golden brown and muffin tests done.

Per serving: (using reduced sugar jam) 197 calories, 4.5 g protein, 35.5 g carbohydrate, 5 g fat, .5 g saturated fat, 1 mg cholesterol, 3 g fiber, 260 mg sodium. Calories from fat: 23 percent. 1.5 grams omega-3 fatty acids.

 ## Flaxseed Focaccia

This recipe calls for fresh rosemary (or dried) in the dough. If you don't care for rosemary, just leave it out. You probably won't notice the flaxseed in this bread—it is fragrant, moist, and delicious! Cut the focaccia into servings and freeze in a resealable bag. When you need some, just thaw a serving or two in the microwave. (For bread machines.)

Makes 8 servings. (Each serving will make a sandwich.)
Dough:

- 1 1/3 cups water
- 1 Tbs. fresh rosemary leaves, finely chopped or 1 1/2 tsp. dried rosemary leaves

- 2 tsp. salt
- 3 tsp. olive oil
- 1/2 cup cornmeal
- 2 3/4 cups unbleached white flour
- 1/3 cup ground flaxseed
- 1 packet (3 tsp.) fast-acting yeast

Topping:

- 3 Tbs. olive oil
- 1 Tbs. garlic, chopped or minced
- 1 Tbs. fresh basil leaves, finely chopped
- 1/4 tsp. salt (optional)
- 1/4 cup parmesan cheese, shredded

1. Add all the dough ingredients, in order, into the bread machine pan. Set for "dough" and press "Start." Check dough after five minutes and add water, a teaspoon at a time, if necessary, to make a smooth, soft ball of dough.

2. In the meantime, blend olive oil, garlic, basil leaves, and salt (if desired) in a small bowl. Set mixture aside.

3. When dough is ready (about 1 hour and 40 minutes) preheat oven to 425 degrees and make sure rack is in the center position. Sprinkle a heavy baking sheet with extra cornmeal.

4. Remove the dough from the machine to a lightly floured work surface. Pat dough into a 1-inch thick round or square. Place it on the prepared baking sheet and poke dimples all over the surface of the dough with your fingertips. Cover with a clean towel and allow to rise on or near oven as it warms up for about 30 minutes.

5. Spread the oil mixture over the top and sprinkle with shredded parmesan cheese.

6. Bake focaccia for 10 minutes, then reduce heat to 350 degrees. Bake about 10-12 minutes more, or until top is golden.

Use as a side dish or as the bread for a gourmet sandwich.

Per serving: 314 calories, 8 g protein, 42.5 g carbohydrate, 12 g fat, 2 g saturated fat, 2 mg cholesterol, 3 g fiber, 593 mg sodium. Calories from fat: 35 percent. 1.7 grams omega-3 fatty acids.

 ## Flaxseed Maple Scones

If you even barely like the taste of maple, you will find these scones addicting! I even adjusted the recipe for a food processor to make these scones a cinch to make. These scones are loaded with ground flaxseed, so 1 scone will give you a day's supply of flaxseed. They freeze well in plastic resealable bags. You can even eat them right out of the freezer!

Makes 8 scones.

Scones:
- 1 1/2 cups all-purpose flour
- 1/3 cup oats
- 1/2 cup ground flaxseed
- 2 Tbs. sugar
- 1/2 tsp. salt
- 1 Tbs. baking powder
- 2 Tbs. maple syrup
- 2 Tbs. canola oil
- 1 egg
- 1/2 cup whole milk (low-fat milk will work too)
- 1/2 tsp. maple extract (3/4 tsp. if you prefer a stronger maple flavor)
- 2/3 cup pecans coarsely chopped (a little smaller than "pecan pieces" but bigger than "finely chopped" pecans)
- Canola cooking spray

Maple Glaze:
- 1 1/2 cups powdered sugar
- 1/2 tsp. maple extract
- 5 tsp. water

1. Preheat oven to 425 degrees. Make an 8-inch circle with canola cooking spray on a thick baking sheet.

2. Add flour, oats, flaxseed, sugar, salt, and baking powder to food processor bowl. Pulse to mix and finely grind the oats with the flour.

3. Add maple syrup and canola oil to the flour mixture and pulse to blend well.

4. In a separate small bowl, beat the egg lightly with the milk and 1/2 tsp. maple extract. Pour the milk mixture into the flour mixture in the food processor. Pulse briefly to make a dough.

5. Place dough on well floured surface. Sprinkle pecans over the top and knead lightly 4 times to evenly distribute the pecans. Pat dough into a 7 1/2-inch circle. Cut into 8 wedges. Place wedges in a circle on prepared baking sheet. Bake in center of oven for about 13-15 minutes (top will be lightly browned).

6. While scones are baking, add glaze ingredients to a small bowl and stir well until smooth. Remove scones from oven to wire rack and let cool about three to five minutes. Spread glaze generously over each scone. Once glaze has dried (about 15 minutes) the scones can be served! They keep well overnight in a resealable plastic bag.

Per serving: 330 calories, 6 g protein, 51 g carbohydrate, 12 g fat, 4 g fiber, 38 mg cholesterol, 370 mg sodium. Calories from fat: 33 percent. 1.3 grams omega-3 fatty acids.

Note: Because the fat grams mainly come from the pecans and the canola oil, most of the fat is the preferred monounsaturated fat!

Best bean recipes

 ## High-Legume Fried Rice

Makes 4 servings.
- 3 Tbs. canola oil
- 1/4 cup green onions, sliced, firmly packed
- 3/4 cup frozen green peas
- 3/4 cup boiled or canned soy beans (Some super-markets carry "boiled soy beans in pod" in the freezer section.) If using frozen, follow the directions on the bag to finish cooking, then remove the soy beans from the pods.
- 1/2 cup diced lean ham (optional)
- 4 cups cooked steamed rice
- 1 egg beaten with 1/4 cup egg substitute
- 1/2 tsp. salt
- 1 to 2 Tbs. light or regular soy sauce

1. Heat oil in wok or large nonstick saucepan to very hot. Add green onion and let sit for one minute.
2. Add green peas, soy beans, ham (if desired), and rice. Let stand for a minute.
3. Push away the mixture toward the edges of the pan, leaving the middle of the pan open, and pour in the egg mixture.
4. Let sit for about 20 seconds, then begin to stir the eggs for another 20 seconds.
5. Stir fry the entire mixture together for a couple of minutes, sprinking salt and soy sauce over the top. Add more soy sauce at table if desired.

Per serving: (with 2 Tbs. light soy sauce) 448 calories, 14.5 g protein, 64 g carbohydrate, 14 g fat, 1.5 g saturated fat, 53 mg cholesterol, 6 g fiber, 590 mg sodium. Calories from fat: 28 percent.

The 3-Minute Burrito

Makes 1 burrito.

- 1/2 cup cooked or canned pinto beans or pinquitos (small brown beans), drained and rinsed
- 1 Tbs. chopped fresh cilantro (optional)
- 2 Tbs. light or fat-free sour cream
- 1 green onion, chopped
- 1/8 cup chunky salsa (mild or hot, depending on preference)
- 1 burrito-size flour tortilla
- 1 1/2 ounces reduced-fat Monterey Jack or sharp cheddar cheese, grated (about a heaping 1/3 cup)

1. In small bowl, toss beans, cilantro, sour cream, green onion, and salsa together.
2. Heat tortilla in microwave on a double thickness of paper towel for about 1 minute or until soft.
3. Sprinkle cheese evenly over the tortilla.
4. Spread bean mixture in center of tortilla. Fold bottom and top ends of tortilla in and roll up into a burrito.
5. Microwave 1 more minute or until burrito is heated through.

Per serving: 430 calories, 23.5 g protein, 53.5 g carbohydrate, 14.5 g fat, 7 grams saturated fat, 26 mg cholesterol, 6 g fiber, 480 mg sodium. Calories from fat: 30 percent.

 Pintos and Cheese

Makes 1 serving.

- 1/2 cup fat-free or vegetarian refried beans
- 2 Tbs. salsa (or 1 tsp. chili sauce) or to taste

- 1 ounce reduced-fat Monterey Jack cheese, grated

1. Spread half of beans in microwave-safe serving bowl. Top beans with half of the salsa.

2. In small bowl, toss grated cheese with green onion. Sprinkle half of cheese and onion mixture over beans.

3. Spread remaining beans over the top then add remaining salsa.

4. Sprinkle remaining cheese and onion over the top.

5. Microwave on high for 2 to 3 minutes or until cheese bubbles.

Per serving: 215 calories, 12 g protein, 29.5 g carbohydrate, 6 g fat, 3 g saturated fat, 15 mg cholesterol, 7 g fiber, 750 mg sodium. Calories from fat: 25 percent.

 ## Quick-Fix Chili and Fries

Makes 2 servings.

- 12 ounces low-fat frozen french fries (Ore-Ida Country Fries or Steak Fries)

- 2 oz. reduced-fat sharp cheddar, grated (about 1/2 cup firmly packed)

- 15 ounces vegetarian canned chili (Hormel brand works well)

1. Preheat oven to 450 degrees. Arrange frozen french fries in a single layer on baking sheet or shallow pan. Bake 20 to 25 minutes, turning after 15 minutes, or until desired crispness and color.

2. Spoon chili into two serving bowls. Heat in microwave (about 3 minutes for each bowl, on high) or place in a small casserole dish and heat in oven along with the french fries.

3.   Sprinkle grated cheese over the chili before serving.
      Serve with fries on the side.

Per serving: 500 calories, 25 g protein, 77 g carbohydrate,
10 g fat, 3 g saturated fat, 20 mg cholesterol, 13 g fiber, 1,080
mg sodium. Calories from fat: 18 percent.

Breakfast ideas

I know this looks like it takes a bit of time, what with
whipping egg whites and everything—but once you know
what you're doing, you can turn this out in 10 minutes. If
you don't want to whip the egg whites, just beat them into
the rest of the egg mixture (it won't be as fluffy, but it still
tastes great).

 ## Light Denver Omelette for Two

Makes 2 servings.
- Canola cooking spray
- 1 cup sliced fresh mushrooms (or other
  vegetable)
- 1 medium green pepper, chopped
- 4 green onions, sliced diagonally
- 1/4 tsp. dried basil
- 1/2 cup chicken broth (water can also
  be used)
- 3 ounces (1/2 cup slightly heaping) lean ham,
  cut into 2-inch long strips
- 1/2 cup cherry tomatoes, halved (or other
  tomatoes)
- 1/2 cup egg substitute
- 2 eggs, separated

1. Coat a medium nonstick frying pan with canola cooking spray, and heat over medium heat. Add mushrooms, green pepper, green onions, and basil. Sauté about 30 seconds, then pour in the chicken broth and cook, stirring frequently, until vegetables are tender. Stir in ham and cherry tomatoes and cook about a minute to heat through.

2. Blend egg substutute and egg yolks in medium-sized bowl and set aside. With mixer, beat egg whites until stiff. Carefully fold egg whites into egg-yolk mixture.

3. Coat a nonstick omelette pan or small nonstick frying pan with canola cooking spray (or use 1/2 tsp. canola oil or canola margarine), and heat over medium-low heat. Spread half of egg mixture in pan. Heat until top looks firm (about 2 minutes). If your pan cooks hotter than normal (as some nonstick pans do), cook over low heat. Flip omelette over to lightly brown other side (about 1 minute).

4. Fill with half of the vegetable-ham filling, and fold as desired. Remove to serving plate. Repeat with remaining egg mixture to make 2 fluffy omelettes.

Per serving: 190 calories, 9 g carbohydrate, 22 g protein, 7 g fat, 2 g saturated fat, 229 mg cholesterol, 2 g fiber, 690 mg sodium. Calories from fat: 35 percent.

 # Egg Muffin Sandwich Lite

Makes 2 sandwiches.
- 2 English muffins, toasted
- 1 egg

- 1/4 cup egg substitute
- 2 slices Canadian bacon (or thick slices lean ham)
- 1 6.5-oz empty tuna can (or similar), washed, labels removed
- Freshly-ground pepper
- 2 slices 1/3 low-fat American cheese slices (or similar)
- Canola cooking spray

1. Coat half of a 9-inch nonstick frying pan with canola cooking spray, and heat over medium heat.

2. In small bowl, beat the egg with egg substitute; set aside.

3. Place Canadian bacon in the pan over the spray coated area. Spray inside of tuna can with canola cooking spray, and set can on the other side of the pan to start heating. When bottom side of the bacon is light brown, flip over to the other side and cook until light brown. Remove slices from pan and set aside.

4. Pour half of egg mixture (1/4 cup) into tuna can. Sprinkle with freshly ground pepper to taste. When the surface of egg begins to firm, cut around the inside of the can with a butter knife to free the edges. Turn the egg over with a cake fork, and cook 1 minute more.

5. Remove egg from can.

6. Coat can with canola cooking spray. Repeat with remaining egg.

7. To assemble, layer English muffin bottom with a slice of cheese, then egg, a piece of Canadian bacon, and the English muffin top. To reheat, microwave each sandwich for 20 seconds on high.

Per serving: 287 calories, 21.5 g protein, 30.5 g carbohydrate, 9 g fat, 3.8 g saturated fat, 130 mg cholesterol, 1.5 g fiber, 1100 mg sodium. Calories from fat: 28 percent.

Sun-Dried Tomato Pesto Bagel Spread

Makes spread for about 3 bagels.

- 1/2 cup light cream cheese
- 1 clove garlic, minced or pressed
- 2 tsp. basil leaves, bottled in water, fresh/chopped, or dried soaked in warm water
- 2 tsp. julienne-style sun-dried tomatoes from bag, soaked in warm water until tender, then drain
- Pine nuts, pecans, or walnuts

1. Add all ingredients to small food processor and process until well blended. Spread on bagels.

Per serving: (with plain bagel) 300 calories, 40.5 g carbohydrate, 14 g protein, 9 g fat, 4.5 g saturated fat, 20 mg cholesterol, 1 g fiber*, 205 mg sodium. Calories from fat: 27 percent. *Using a whole-grain bagel will add about 3 g of fiber per serving.

The Lox-ness Monster Bagel Spread

Makes about 1/2 cup of spread (enough for about 4 bagels).

- 1/2 cup light cream cheese
- 2 ounces lox, finely chopped
- 1 green onion, finely chopped
- Pinch of fresh or dried dill (optional)
- Pinch of capers (optional)

Blend all ingredients in food processor until well mixed. You should still be able to see some small pieces of lox. Spread on bagels.

Per serving: (with plain bagel) 270 calories, 13 g protein, 38.5 g carbohydrate, 7 g fat, 3.5 g saturated fat, 18 mg cholesterol, 1 g fiber*, 560 mg sodium. Calories from fat: 23 percent.
* Using a whole-grain bagel will add about 3 grams of fiber per serving.

 ## Apple Lover's Oatmeal

Makes 1 serving.
- 1 packet instant oatmeal, plain. (If you use flavored, sweetened instant oatmeal, such as "maple & brown sugar," then don't add the brown sugar.)
- 1 individual serving applesauce (3.9 oz), unsweetened (1/3 cup)
- 2 Tbs. brown sugar
- 1/4 tsp. ground cinnamon
- 1/2 cup low-fat milk (or similar—soy milk or almond milk can also be used)
- In a large microwave-safe soup bowl, blend all ingredients together. Microwave on high for 1 1/2 minutes. Stir, then microwave for another 1 1/2 minutes. Serve hot.

Per serving: 225 calories, 5.5 g protein, 47 g carbohydrate, 2 grams fat, .8 g saturated fat, 5 mg cholesterol, 2.5 g fiber, 140 mg sodium. Calories from fat: 8 percent.

Note: To make a more balanced breakfast, enjoy this oatmeal with a strip or two of Louis Rich turkey bacon.

Scrumptious side dishes

 ## Monounsaturated Side Salad

This salad is not just rich in monounsaturated fats—it's rich in fiber.

Makes 4 servings.

* 1/2 avocado, cut into bite-size pieces
* 1/2 cucumber, sliced
* 1 cup chopped tomatoes or cherry tomatoes cut in half
* 1 cup kidney beans (or 1/2 cup kidney beans and 1/2 cup garbanzo), drained and rinsed
* 6 Tbs. Wish-Bone olive oil vinaigrette (or other dressing that uses olive oil or canola oil)
* 4 to 6 cups ready-to-serve salad greens of your choice

1. Place avocado, cucumber, tomatoes, and beans into a serving bowl. Toss with dressing; set aside in refrigerator until needed.
2. Right before mealtime, toss vegetable mixture with lettuce.

Per serving: 155 calories, 6 g protein, 19 g carbohydrate, 7 g fat, .7 g saturated fat, 0 mg cholesterol, 7 g fiber, 460 mg sodium. Calories from fat: 43 percent.

Easy 3-Bean Salad

Makes 4 servings.

- 1 8.75-ounce can kidney beans, drained and rinsed (about 1 cup)
- 1 8.75-ounce can garbanzo beans, drained and rinsed (about 1 cup)
- 1 8.75-ounce can green or yellow wax beans, drained and rinsed (about 1 cup)
- 1/4 cup finely diced yellow or white onion
- 4 Tbs. bottled vinaigrette (that uses olive oil or canola oil)

Add all ingredients to serving bowl. Toss well. This will store covered in the refrigerator for several days.

Per serving: 160 calories, 7 g protein, 27.5 g carbohydrate, 3 g fat, 0 g saturated fat, 0 mg cholesterol, 7 g fiber, 635 mg sodium. Calories from fat: 17 percent.

Quick snacks and pick-me-ups

 Quick Ranch Dip (With Vegetables)

Makes about 1/4 cup of dip.

- 1 tsp. Hidden Valley Ranch Dip powder
- 1/4 cup light or nonfat sour cream
- 1 tsp. canola mayonnaise (if available), otherwise use regular
- Assorted raw vegetables for dipping (baby carrots, celery sticks, broccoli and cauliflower florets)
1. Combine all dip ingredients in a small bowl. Stir well with spoon.
2. Serve with assorted vegetables.

Per serving: (1/8 cup dip with 1 cup raw vegetables) 95 calories, 3 g protein, 16.5 g carbohydrate, 2 g fat, .2 g saturated fat, 1 mg cholesterol, 3.3 g fiber, 325 mg sodium. Calories from fat: 19 percent.

Spicy Hummus with Crudites and Crackers

This is a variation on the really tasty Middle Eastern dip/spread. You may have to search a bit to find tahini, although it is available in many supermarkets on the East and West Coasts.

Makes about 3 cups of dip.

- 2 15-oz. cans 50% less sodium garbanzo beans
- 3 cloves garlic, minced or pressed
- 1/3 cup tahini (sesame seed paste)
- 1/4 cup lemon juice
- 3 Tbs. light or fat-free sour cream
- 2 Tbs. light cream cheese
- 1/4 tsp. seasoning salt (optional)
- 1/4 tsp. ground cumin
- 1/4 tsp. paprika
- 2 Tbs. finely chopped fresh parsley (optional)
- Crudites: choose crisp vegetables like red bell pepper, carrots, celery, cauliflower, broccoli, green beans, etc.
- Crackers: choose from many reduced-fat crackers on the market.

1. Drain garbanzo beans and rinse well. (Reserve some of the liquid to add back if you need it to make a thinner dip.)
2. Place beans, garlic, tahini, lemon juice, sour cream, cream cheese, seasoning salt, cumin, paprika, and parsley in food processor. Blend

until somewhat smooth. Add more lemon juice or garbanzo liquid to taste. Use immediately or cover and refrigerate (will keep for several days). Serve with vegetables and crackers.

Per serving: (1/3 cup dip) 100 calories, 1 g protein, 9 g carbohydrate, 5.5 g fat, 1 g saturated fat, 1 mg cholesterol, 3 g fiber, 120 mg sodium. Calories from fat: 50 percent.

When each serving is eaten with a cup of suggested vegetables, the fiber increases to about 6 grams a serving.

 ## Iced Café Mocha

This is a great drink to slip 2 teaspoons of ground flaxseed into. If you want to use the reduced-sugar chocolate syrup, go ahead, but I personally don't care for the flavor.
Makes 1 drink.

- 4 ice cubes
- 2 level tsp. instant espresso powder (available in coffee section of most supermarkets)
- 1 cup 1-percent or 2-percent low-fat milk
- 2 Tbs. chocolate syrup

1. Place ice cubes in blender or food processor and pulse until crushed.
2. In small cup blend espresso powder with 2 Tbs. of the milk. Add to blender along with remaining milk and chocolate syrup.
3. Pulse until nicely blended. Pour into cup and enjoy!

Per serving: 185 calories, 9 g protein, 31 g carbohydrate, 3 g fat, 1.6 g saturated fat, 10 mg cholesterol, 1 g fiber, 165 mg sodium. Calories from fat: 15 percent.

Oatmeal Raisin Bites

You can make a batch of these babies, then pop them in the freezer in a resealable plastic bag. Take out a cookie whenever you need one. They thaw quickly in the microwave or at room temperature.

Makes 32 large cookies.

- 6 Tbs. canola margarine or butter, softened
- 6 Tbs. fat-free or light cream cheese
- 1 cup packed brown sugar
- 1/2 cup granulated sugar
- 1/4 cup low-fat buttermilk
- 1/4 cup egg substitute
- 2 Tbs. maple syrup
- 2 Tbs. vanilla extract
- 1 cup unbleached flour
- 1/2 tsp. baking soda
- 1 1/2 tsp. ground cinnamon
- 1/4 tsp. salt
- 2 cups quick or old fashioned oats
- 1 cup raisins
- 1/2 cup chopped walnuts (optional)

1. Preheat oven to 350 degrees. Coat two cookie sheets with canola cooking spray. In a large bowl, beat the butter with cream cheese. Beat in the sugars, buttermilk, egg substitute, maple syrup, and vanilla. Beat until light and fluffy.

2. Combine the flour, baking soda, cinnamon, and salt; beat into the butter mixture.

3. Stir in the oats, raisins, and nuts if desired, mixing well.

4. Use a cookie scoop (or drop by rounded table-spoonfuls) to form cookies and place 2 inches apart on the prepared cookie sheets. For flatter (rather than rounded) cookies, press each cookie mound down lightly with a spoon, spatula, or your fingers.

5. Bake one cookie sheet at a time, in the upper third of oven for about 10 minutes, or until lightly browned. Remove the cookies to wire racks to cool completely. Store in an airtight container.

Per serving: 120 calories, 2 g protein, 22 g carbohydrate, 3 g fat, .4 g saturated fat, 5 mg cholesterol, 1.2 g fiber, 36 mg sodium. Calories from fat: 22 percent.

Quick omega-3 entrées

 ## Lemon Dijon Salmon

Makes 2 servings.
*   2 salmon steaks (about 6 ounces each)
*   1 Tbs. Dijon mustard
*   Garlic salt (about 1/2 tsp.)
*   Freshly-ground pepper
*   1/2 onion, thinly sliced
*   1/2 lemon
*   2 to 3 tsp. capers

1. Preheat oven to 400 degrees. Line a 9-inch pie plate with a large sheet of foil (enough so it can be wrapped back over the fish and sealed) and spray foil generously with canola cooking spray. Lay salmon steaks in prepared pan.

2. Spread fish steaks evenly with Dijon mustard.

3. Sprinkle fish steaks with garlic salt and ground pepper to your liking.

4. Lay thinly sliced onion over the top.

5. Squeeze 1/2 lemon over the top of the salmon and sprinkle capers over the top.

6. Wrap edges of foil over the top of fish and seal edges together. Bake about 15 minutes. Open foil and let bake about 5 minutes more or until salmon is cooked throughout.

7. Serve with steamed rice or cooked pasta and some vegetables.

Per serving: 231 calories, 30 g protein, 5 g carbohydrate, 10 g fat, 1.5 g saturated fat, 80 mg cholesterol, 1 g fiber, 678 mg sodium. Calories from fat: 39 percent.

Per serving: (when each serving is served with 3/4 cup steamed rice and a cup of broccoli) 475 calories, 38.5 g protein, 56 g carbohydrate, 11 g fat, 1.7 g saturated fat, 80 mg cholesterol, 6.5 g fiber, 720 mg sodium. Calories from fat: 21 percent. 1.5 grams omega-3 fatty acids.

 Simple Salmon Pasta Salad

This is one of my favorite salads. I make extra grilled salmon on purpose so I can make this salad the next day with the leftovers.

Makes about 2 entrée servings.

Salmon:

• 2 cups bow tie or rotelle pasta made with semolina flour, cooked al dente

• 1 cup salmon flakes (freshly cooked or grilled salmon fillets or steaks, broken into flakes with fork, with no bones or skin)

- 1 cup crisp-tender asparagus pieces, steamed or microwaved
- 3 green onions, finely chopped

Dressing:

- 1 Tbs. canola mayonnaise (if available otherwise use regular)
- 2 Tbs. fat-free or light sour cream
- 1 Tbs. lemon juice
- 1 1/2 tsp. Dijon or prepared mustard
- 1/2 tsp. dill weed
- Black pepper to taste

1. Place pasta, salmon, asparagus, and green onions in serving bowl.
2. Blend dressing ingredients in a 1- or 2-cup measure until smooth. Add to pasta salad ingredients and stir to mix.

Per serving: 339 calories, 18 g protein, 45 g carbohydrate, 9.5 g fat, 1.5 g saturated fat, 29 mg cholesterol, 3 g fiber, 122 mg sodium. Calories from fat: 26 percent. 1 g omega-3 fatty acid per serving.

 Easy Omega-3 Fatty Acid Tuna Sandwich

- 6 1/2 ounces albacore tuna, canned in spring water, drained
- 1 Tbs. sweet or dill pickle relish (optional)
- 1/4 tsp. salt (optional)
- 1 Tbs. canola mayonnaise (or regular)
- 1/2 Tbs. minced onion
- 1/4 cup minced celery

- 1 Tbs. light or fat-free sour cream
- Pepper to taste
- 2 slices whole wheat or whole grain bread (toasted if desired)
- Lettuce leaves and tomato slices
1. Combine tuna, relish, salt, mayo, sour cream, onion, and celery in small bowl; mix well. Add pepper to taste.
2. Spread mixture on slices of bread to make a sandwich. Add lettuce leaves, and tomato slices.

Per serving: 320 calories, 27 g protein, 34 g carbohydrate, 1.4 g saturated fat, 27 mg cholesterol, 4.5 g fiber, 676 mg sodium. Calories from fat: 25 percent. About 0.5 omega-3 fatty acids from tuna and about 0.5 from the canola mayonnaise.

Other quick entrées

 Oat Bran Meat Loaf

This meat loaf tastes so much better than it sounds. Each serving contributes 5 grams of mostly soluble fiber to the meal too!

Makes 5 servings

- 1 1/4 cup canned chick-peas (garbanzo beans), drained and rinsed
- 1/2 cup oat bran
- 1/2 tsp. black pepper
- 1/2 tsp. salt (optional)
- 2 cloves garlic, minced or pressed, or 1/2 teaspoon garlic powder
- 1 Tbs. Worcestershire sauce

- 2 Tbs. Heinz chili sauce
- 1 Tbs. prepared mustard
- 1 lb. ground sirloin (about 9-percent fat)
- 1 cup grated, reduced-fat, sharp cheddar cheese (optional)
- 1 small onion, finely chopped
- Canola cooking spray
- 1 cup tomato sauce

1. Preheat oven to 350 degrees. Coat a 9-by-5-inch loaf pan with canola cooking spray.

2. Add ingredients up to and including mustard to mixer or food processor. You can also mash with pastry blender or potato masher.

3. Process until well mixed (there will still be some lumps).

4. If using a mixer, add beef, cheese, and onion to bean mixture and mix until well blended. If using a food processor, blend bean mixture with beef, cheese, and onion with hands (or use a spoon) in a large mixing bowl.

5. Add mixture to pan and form into a loaf.

6. Bake 30 minutes. Pour tomato sauce over the top and bake 15 minutes longer.

Per serving: 286 calories, 24.5 g protein, 28.5 g carbohydrate, 10 g fat, 3.5 g saturated fat, 33 mg cholesterol, 5 g fiber, 700 mg sodium. Calories from fat: 29 percent.

Light Club Sandwich

Makes 1 sandwich.

- 2 slices Louis Rich turkey bacon (or similar)
- 2 slices whole wheat bread
- 1 tsp. canola mayonnaise (or regular) blended with 1 tsp. of light or fat-free sour cream
- 2 lettuce leaves
- 1 large slice turkey breast (about 2 ounces)
- Pepper to taste
- 1/2 large tomato, sliced

1. Cook bacon in nonstick frying pan, over low heat, until crisp.

2. Spread one side of each bread slice lightly with mayonnaise mixture. Arrange lettuce leaf on one slice; top with one slice of turkey; sprinkle with pepper, then cover with another bread slice, mayonnaise side up. Top with another leaf of lettuce, tomato slices, bacon slices, and remaining bread slice, mayonnaise side down.

3. Cut sandwich diagonally into fourths; secure each quarter with decorated toothpicks if desired.

Per serving: 350 calories, 19 g protein, 38 g carbohydrate, 12.5 g fat, 2.7 g saturated fat, 49 mg cholesterol, 5.5 g fiber, 1,400 mg sodium. Calories from fat: 32 percent.

Chapter 6

Navigating the Supermarket

I t's easy to get confused while shopping in the trenches (a.k.a. your typical grocery store). Each product label your eye catches inevitably hits you with countless advertising slogans and nutrition terms. Just remember the bottom line is that all these companies are basically trying to sell you something—they all want a piece of your food budget. The package might boast "sugar-free" or "fat-free" but it's the nutrition information label that's going to tell you whether that product has just as many grams of carbohydrate or just as many calories as the regular products.

It's also the nutrition information label that is going to confess what the company considers the serving size to be. A single serving of Snickers is 1/2 of a 2-ounce bar. A serving of most ice creams is usually 1/2 cup. A serving of some of the cookie brands is 1 while the serving of many pot pies is 1/2 a pot pie. The serving size of many individual or small frozen pizzas is 1/3 of the "small" pizza. There are some reduced-fat ice cream bars out there that, when you check the label, still contain more than 13 grams of fat per serving. The moral of this story is—read your labels. The more you know about the product, the better off you will be.

How to speak supermarket-ese

Here are the definitions of some of the labeling or advertising terms that you might be most interested in:

Free means that a product contains no or only negligible amounts of fat, saturated fat, cholesterol, sodium, sugar, and/or calories.

"Percent fat free" is used only on low-fat or fat-free products. The term is a reflection of the amount of the food's weight that is fat free. For example, if a serving of food weighs 100 grams and two of the grams come from fat; it can be called "98 percent fat free."

Low means different things in different circumstances:

- Low calorie: 40 calories or fewer per serving.
- Low-fat: 3 grams or fewer per serving.
- Low saturated fats: no more than 1 gram per serving.
- Low cholesterol: fewer than 20 milligrams per serving.
- Low sodium: fewer than 140 milligrams per serving.

Reduced lets the customer know that a product has been nutritionally altered and contains 25 percent less of a nutrient or of calories than the regular product.

Light (Lite) means the product contains 50 percent less fat (in grams) than the regular product or the calories have been reduced by at least 1/3 of what they were in the regular product. Light can also be used to refer to the texture and color of a food; however, the label must spell this out (for example, light brown sugar).

Daily values on nutrition labels show how a food fits into the overall daily diet. The daily values are based on a daily diet of 2,000 calories (individuals are supposed to adjust the values to fit their own calorie intake). The daily values provide figures for fat, saturated fat, cholesterol, sodium, carbohydrates, fiber, vitamins and minerals.

A sugar by any other name

Sugars or sweeteners can go by many names other than "sugar." Other names for sugar that you might see on an ingredient label are:

- Sucrose.
- High fructose corn syrup.
- Fructose.
- Brown sugar.
- Maltose.
- Corn sweeteners.
- Dextrose.
- Honey.
- Syrups (such as corn syrup, maple syrup, or molasses).

Don't let all this confuse you too much, you'll get the information you need for counting and calculating in the nutrition information label—grams of total carbohydrate per serving. (Make sure to check out the serving size—it might surprise you.)

Supermarket 101

There are several lessons to be learned before navigating the supermarket—with or without diabetes. The first is to look to the label—check the portion size, the grams of fat, carbohydrates, and calories when shopping for and comparing food products.

The second lesson is a bit more difficult to master. Some of us may be using these fat-free products as an excuse to overeat. I don't think we are entirely to blame here. If these products aren't as satisfying, we're probably more likely to keep on eating and eating in the hope of reaching some level of satisfaction. Also, some of the advertising has basically encouraged us to eat as much as we want—after all, it's fat-free! So select light and fat-free products that you truly like—that taste satisfying to you—that you can eat in modest serving sizes. Otherwise, they aren't going to do a hill of beans for your health and enjoyment.

For example, I really love Cracker Barrel Light Sharp Cheddar; it is real cheese to me. My family has Louis Rich turkey bacon and we don't miss real bacon. Reduced-fat Bisquick is a staple in my house. We all think Louis Rich turkey franks and Ball Park Lite franks taste terrific. These are the types of products you want to keep buying—the ones that you truly enjoy.

Last, but not least, figure the grams of carbohydrate into your daily eating plan.

You will also quickly learn, when sampling some of the new fat-free or sugar-free products, that some companies have definitely gone too far. In my opinion, certain foods simply aren't meant to be fat-free. If you take all the fat out of a food that was mostly fat to begin with, such as mayonnaise, cheese, or butter, then what have you really got? Something other than mayonnaise, cheese, or butter—that's for sure. It's not fat-free butter; it's just a new kind of yellow goop.

More than half of the new fat-free, sugar-free, or light products I try end up in the garbage can. But the upside is that about 20 percent (or one in five) of the products are keepers. A number of products have successfully hit their optimal level of fat. These are the foods that withstood a modest reduction in fat without a huge loss in taste satisfaction. You'll find them listed in this chapter.

Avoiding the land mines

Have you ever noticed that the nutrition facts information on the label of a baking mix or cake mix is listed in two columns: Mix and Baked (or As Prepared)? Normally they will give you two amounts of fat grams; one from the mix and one for the total amount of fat per serving after it is prepared. This is important information, because many of these mixes call for 1/3 cup of oil, three eggs, or a stick of butter.

Several companies have started giving only the grams of fat in the mix. If you look real closely, which is what I get paid to do, you'll see a tiny asterisk next to the grams of fat. Then you look down at the very bottom of the label and in small print it reads something like this: "Amount in mix."

They do give you the percent daily value for grams of fat "as prepared," but let's face it, what does that really mean to most people. Most people just quickly scan the label until they see grams of fat. I can just picture people thinking, "Oh, goody, 4 grams of fat!" When in reality, if they follow the directions on the box, a serving has something more like 9 or 13 grams of fat per serving.

Just so you know what to watch out for—here is an example:

Pillsbury Thick 'n Fudgy Cheesecake Swirl Deluxe Brownie Mix: A serving of mix contains 4.5 grams of fat. When you follow the directions on the box, adding 1/4 cup oil and 2 eggs to the mix, the grams of fat per serving increases to 9 grams of fat. But you won't see 9 grams anywhere on the label. If you look really hard you'll find 14 percent daily value for fat in the "prepared" column. You have to do a little math to get to 9 from the 14 percent daily value given on the label.

F.Y.I. A little math lesson...

If you look at the percent daily value guide at the very bottom of the label (in smaller print), you'll see "less than 65 grams of fat" listed for a 2,000-calorie standard intake. Now multiply 65 grams by 14 percent and you get 9 grams of fat.

It's all in a name

We've come to rely on certain brands with diet-sounding names to steer us toward the better choices where our waistlines and diabetes are concerned. Weight Watchers, Lean Cuisine, and Slim Fast, for example, are all music to the ears. But don't let those seductive names fool you. Some of these products are just as high in calories, fat, and carbohydrate grams as the overtly "sinful" products farther down the aisle.

In many cases, what they are selling you is portion control and a pretty name (for a handsome price). The Nestle Sweet Success Peanut Butter snack bar weighs in at 31 grams with 100 calories, 3.5 grams of fat, and 23 grams of carbohydrate. Now jog just a few feet farther and you'll find Kudos Peanut Butter bar with 130 calories, 5 grams fat, and less carbohydrate—19 grams.

But at least it's not like eating a candy bar, right? Wrong. Twenty-eight grams of Milky Way (1/2 of a regular-sized bar) actually contains almost the same amount of calories (118) and fat (4 grams) as the Slim Fast and Nestle Sweet Success snack bars.

Fat-free, but full of calories

Here's a news flash—just because a product is fat-free doesn't mean it is calorie-free or that you can eat the whole box in one sitting. In fact, many of these fat-free products have just as many calories as the full-fat versions. How can that be? In a word—sugar. Sugar, whether it comes from honey, corn syrup, brown sugar, or high fructose corn syrup, can add moisture and help tenderize bakery products. When added to foods like ice cream, it adds flavor and structure. So I'm not surprised that manufacturers have turned to sugar for assistance while developing reduced-fat and fat-free products.

The majority of the fat-free and lower-fat products on the supermarket shelves only offer us average savings of 10 or 20 calories per serving. Does this mean we shouldn't buy any of these products? No—this means to truly benefit from these lower-fat or fat-free products, we need to watch our serving size and keep track of the grams of carbohydrates we are taking in.

Taking a tour of your supermarket

I walked around my supermarket, pen and paper in hand, with an eye for foods and products that someone like you might want to know about. I looked for:

- Lower-carbohydrate and reduced-calorie products that might come in handy when you are trying to balance a meal or snack.
- Good, easy sources of soluble fiber (and fiber in general).
- Quick sources of omega-3 fatty acids and mono-unsaturated fats.
- Whole-grain products that would contribute fiber and other nutrients, and also possibly have a positive effect on our blood sugars.

- I also included nutrition information for convenience products you might be tempted to buy, so you can make the very best choices.

Frozen breakfast foods

You can buy everything from breakfast muffins to a complete egg, sausage, and hash brown breakfast in the frozen food section. Watch out though—frozen breakfast foods are either brimming with saturated or trans fats or sugar. You've got to keep an eye out for flashy health claims too. There is a popular brand boasting that their "healthy muffins" are fiber-rich, but you can get just as much fiber (and a lot less sugar) from a bowl of Cheerios. I've listed the frozen waffles that contain some fiber and some lighter frozen sausages that might help balance out an otherwise mostly carbohydrate breakfast, and added a few frozen breakfast convenience products that are fairly well balanced between fat, carbohydrates and protein.

Frozen Breakfast Foods

	Cal. (g)	Carbs (g, %*)	Fat (g)	Pro. (g)	Fib. (mg)	Sod. (mg)
Eggo Golden Oat waffles (made w/oat bran), 2	140	26	2.5 (16%)	5	3	270
Eggo Raisin & Bran Waffles, 2	210	36	6 (26%)	5	5	430
Eggo Nutri-Grain Multigrain Waffles, 2	160	29	5 (28%)	5	5	360
Jones Brown & Serve Light (pork and rice links), 2	110	1	9 (73%)	7	0	280
Swift Premium Brown 'N Serve, 3	120	1	9 (67%)	7	0	280
Weight Watchers Smart Ones: English Muffin Sandwich	210	28	5 (21%)	13	2	420
Weight Watchers Smart Ones: Handy Ham & Cheese Omelet	320	30	5 (14%)	13	2	440
Amy's Organic Black Bean Ranchero Breakfast Burrito	230	38	5 (19%)	9	5	480

*Percent of calories from fat

Do you like hash browns?

Do you like hash browns but loathe all the fat the frozen hash browns have? There's a frozen hash brown you can buy that comes with zero fat. You get to decide how much oil to add when you pan fry it, and here's the best part—you decide which oil to fry them in. You can fry them in a little bit of canola oil and make a crispy, tasty hash brown that contributes monounsaturated fat and some omega-3 fatty acids to boot. Take a look:

Ore-Ida Hash Browns: One shredded potato patty contains 70 calories, 0 grams fat and cholesterol, 16 grams carbohydrate, 2 grams protein, 1 gram fiber, and 30 milligrams sodium.

Pan fry 3 of the patties in 1 tablespoon of canola oil (fry for about 6 minutes, turn and fry 4 minutes more). 1 patty contains 110 calories, 4.5 grams fat (3 grams of which are monounsaturated), and 36 percent calories from fat.

Egg substitutes

People with type II diabetes sometimes manage a meal better if it contains some fat (instead of no fat or very low-fat.) So, using all egg substitute (which is fat-free) in meals that are fat-free may not be the best idea. But there are two ways that egg substitutes can be your saving grace:

1. Use egg substitute (which is fat-free) in recipes or meals that are high-fat, to help bring down the total fat to a more moderate level.
2. Use part egg substitutes (which are also cholesterol-free) and part real eggs in baking and cooking to help bring down the cholesterol per serving.

Using egg substitute ups the protein too, because egg substitutes are mostly egg white—the protein portion of the egg. (Remember, all the fat and cholesterol is in the yolk of the egg.) My favorite brand of egg substitute (Egg Beaters) is 99 percent egg white, which explains why it has almost no fat and very few calories. It looks like scrambled eggs, so you can use it in omelets, quiche, and any recipe that calls for beaten eggs. If you use half egg substitute and half real eggs, you will usually have a food or recipe that tastes very similar to the original. For example, if the recipe calls for 4 eggs, you could use 2 eggs and 1/2-cup egg substitute (1/4 cup per egg it replaces).

Egg Substitutes

	Calories	Carbs (g)	Fat (g)	Protein (g)	Sodium (mg)
Egg Beaters	30	1	0	6	125
Scramblers	35	2	0	6	95
All Whites (Papetti Foods)	33	2.5	0	7	100

Like Donuts?

Like donuts? I know I do. Have you tried the Entenmann's light donuts yet? Well, you should. Of course, it isn't something you should eat every breakfast. But if you have a hankering for a donut, this will satisfy, with 50 percent less fat and a few less calories too. Entenmann's offers two variety packs:

The Light Variety Pack, 1 donut contains: 190 calories, 31 grams carbohydrate, 7 grams fat (33 percent calories from fat), 1.5 grams saturated fat, 3 grams protein, 15 milligrams cholesterol, < 1 gram fiber, and 320 milligrams sodium.

The Light Chocolate Lover's Variety Pack, 1 donut contains: 220 calories, 34 grams carbohydrate, 9 grams fat (37 percent calories from fat), 2.5 grams saturated fat, 2 grams protein, 15 milligrams cholesterol, < 1 gram fiber, and 270 milligrams sodium.

Diabetic-friendly frozen entrées

Frozen entrées come in handy in many situations—as a quick lunch and as an easy dinner.

The problem with frozen entrées is that the ones that are lower in fat are almost always too low in calories and carbohydrate and meager in the vegetable department. Many contain around 300 calories, the amount of calories in one measly bagel. In order to make the entrées satisfying, I found myself adding vegetables, cooked rice or noodles, or grated cheese. And if people are eating them as their complete meal, they are also totally devoid of fruit. Most frozen entrées are going to be brimming with sodium. The companies taste-test products with the average American's taste preferences in mind. And the average American likes salt.

You can add an extra 1/2 cup of noodles or rice, 1/2 cup of steamed or frozen vegetables, and a piece or two of fruit to help round out the entrées (which is what I did when I was trying each of the entrées listed on the following page). But this is sort of defeating the purpose of a frozen entree, now isn't it? I listed the nutrition information of some of the frozen entrées I found interesting in my supermarket. For some of the entrées that are begging for some added vegetables and starches, I provided two analysis—one with and one without the added foods.

Because some people with type II diabetes fare better with a little more fat in their meal (preferably monounsaturated fat), I included any non "light" entrée that seemed workable.

Frozen Entrées

	Cal.	Carbs (g)	Fat (g,%*)	Pro. (g)	Fiber (g)	Sod. (mg)
Healthy Choice						
Chicken enchiladas suiza	280	43	6 (19%)	14	5	440
Shrimp & vegetables	270	39	6 (20%)	15	6	580
Herb baked fish	340	54	7 (19%)	16	5	480
Traditional breast of turkey	290	40	4.5 (14%)	22	5	460
Chicken enchilada suprema	300	46	7 (21%)	13	4	560
Lean Cuisine						
Chicken with basil cream sauce	270	35	7 (23%)	16	3	580
Chicken in peanut sauce	290	35	6 (19%)	23	4	590
Baked fish with cheddar shells	270	36	6 (20%)	17	4	540
Fiesta chicken (with black beans, rice, and vegetables)	270	36	5 (17%)	19	4	590
Cheese lasagna with chicken breast scallopini	290	33	8 (25%)	21	3	590
Shrimp and angel hair pasta	290	55	6 (19%)	10	1	590
3-bean chili	250	38	6 (22%)	10	9	590
The Budget Gourmet						
Three cheese lasagna	310	34	12 (35%)	15	2	700
Fettucini and meatballs in wine sauce with green beans	270	40	7 (23%)	15	3	560

Frozen Entrées, continued

	Cal.	Carbs (g)	Fat (g, %*)	Pro. (g)	Fiber (g)	Sod. (mg)
Marie Calender's						
Chili and cornbread	540	67	21 (35%)	21	7	2,110
Sweet and sour chicken	570	86	15 (24%)	23	7	700
Beef tips in mushroom sauce	430	39	17 (36%)	25	6	1,620
Turkey with gravy and dressing	500	52	19 (34%)	31	4	2,040
Spaghetti and meat sauce	670	85	25 (34%)	31	9	1,160
Cheese ravioli in marinara sauce (with garlic bread)	750	96	29 (35%)	25	1	1,070
Stuffed pasta trio	640	40	18 (25%)	15	5	950
Swanson						
Mexican style combination	470	59	18 (34%)	18	5	1,610
Chicken parmigiana	370	40	17 (41%)	13	4	1,010
Herb roasted chicken breast tenders with rice & vegetables	310	4	7 (20%)	16	3	780
Turkey dinner	310	40	8.5	22	5	890

Frozen pizza

I always have a frozen pizza in my freezer for those dinner emergencies that come up every now and then. There are actually a couple of brands out there that aren't too bad on the taste buds—and nutritionally speaking either. Sometimes the serving size on frozen pizza can be a bit optimistic—so make sure you know what that is if you are doing any nutrition calculations. Here are a couple of my favorites:

DiGiorno Four Cheese Pizza: 1/3 of a 12-ounce pizza contains: 280 calories, 34 grams carbohydrate, 9 grams fat (29 percent calories from fat), 5 grams saturated fat, 15 grams protein, 20 milligrams cholesterol, 2 grams fiber, and 700 milligrams sodium.

Wolfgang Puck's Mushroom & Spinach Pizza: 1/2 of a 10.5-ounce pizza contain: 270 calories, 36 grams carbohydrate, 8 grams fat (27 percent calories from fat), 3 grams saturated fat, 14 grams protein, 10 milligrams cholesterol, 5 grams fiber, and 380 milligrams sodium.

Wolfgang Puck's Four Cheese Pizza: 1/2 of a 9.25-ounce pizza contain: 360 calories, 40 grams carbohydrate, 15 grams fat (37 percent calories from fat), 6 grams saturated fat, 17 grams protein, 25 milligrams cholesterol, 5 grams fiber, and 530 milligrams sodium.

Ore-Ida Bagel Bites (Three Cheese): 4 pieces contain: 190 calories, 25 grams carbohydrate, 6 grams fat (28 percent calories from fat), 3.5 grams saturated fat, 9 grams protein, 15 milligrams cholesterol, 1 gram fiber, and 530 milligrams sodium.

Ore-Ida Bagel Bites (Cheese & Pepperoni): 4 pieces contains: 200 calories, 26 grams carbohydrate, 7 grams fat (32 percent calories from fat), 3.5 grams saturated fat, 9 grams protein, 15 milligrams cholesterol, 1 gram fiber, and 610 milligrams sodium.

Lean Pockets (Reduced-Fat) Pepperoni Pizza Deluxe: 1 pocket contains: 270 calories, 37 grams carbohydrate, 7 grams fat (23 percent calories from fat), 2.5 grams saturated fat, 15 grams protein, 35 milligrams cholesterol, 3 grams fiber, and 580 milligrams sodium.

Frozen desserts

I'm one of those people who, if given a nudge or two, could eat ice cream every day. People become addicted to this wonderful multi-season treat with its cold and creamy feeling. It comes in fun flavors, and tops a meal like nothing else. Ice cream needs at least some fat and sugar, or it wouldn't be "ice cream." The following choices are some of the best-tasting "light" options. I included the nutrition information for some of the better sounding sugar-free

Frozen Desserts

	Calories	Carbs.	Fat (%*)
Ice cream			
Dreyer's Grand Light (Edy's Grand Light):			
Rocky Road	120	17	4 (30%)
Mocha Almond Fudge	120	16	5 (37%)
Mint Chocolate Chip	120	17	4 (30%)
Coffee Mousse Crunch	120	18	4 (30%)
French Silk	120	19	4 (30%)
Dreyers (Edy's) No Sugar Added:			
Fat-Free Chocolate Fudge	100	21	0 (0%)
Butter Pecan	110	12	5 (41%)
Vanilla	80	11	3 (34%)
Ice cream Bars: (1 bar)			
Starbucks Frappuccino	110	20	2 (16%)
Nesquik Ice Screamers	100	11	5 (45%)
Tropicana Orange Cream	70	14	1 (13%)
Tropicana Strawberry 'n Cream	70	14	1.5 (19%)
Eskimo Pie Reduced Fat/No Sugar Added—Dark Chocolate Coating	120	13	8 (60%)
Eskimo Pie Reduced Fat/No Sugar Added—Crisp Rice	120	13	8 (60%)
Other:			
Sara Lee Reduced Fat Pound Cake (quarter cake)	280	42	11 (35%)
Weight Watchers Smart Ones: (1 serving)			
New York Style Cheesecake	150	21	5 (30%)
Chocolate Eclair	150	25	4 (24%)

*Percent calories from fat

Most of these items contain per serving about 3 g protein, between 1 and 3 g saturated fat, and about 50 mg sodium, except for the Eskimo Pie (about 6 g sodium) and the Weight Watchers Smart Ones (about 150 mg).

frozen dessert options—but I can't vouch for the flavor. By the way, in case you are curious, 1/2 cup of a "light" ice cream contains about 20 milligrams cholesterol. (We don't include cholesterol in the tables because there are so many other items to list. And, for most people, grams of fat and saturated fat have a greater impact on blood lipids.)

Dairy products

We need milk to keep our cereal company, help liquefy our pancake batter, or lighten our coffee. The great thing about milk is you can take out some of the fat and saturated fat and still have milk that does all the things you want it to do. And as you remove the fat, the cholesterol goes too.

- Milk goes from 35 mg cholesterol in a cup of whole milk down to 15 mg in a cup of 1 percent low-fat milk.

- Cottage cheese goes from 25 mg cholesterol in 1/2 cup of small curd cottage cheese down to 10 mg in low-fat.

- It gets a little tricky with other dairy products. When you take the fat out of cheese, for example, if you start going past the halfway mark, it starts looking and tasting a lot less like cheese and a lot more like plastic.

No matter what the amount of fat, most dairy products should be consumed in reasonable amounts—they all need to be counted into your daily totals, because many contribute carbohydrate grams galore (such as fat-free flavored yogurts). Then, the other dairy products that are low in carbohydrates need to be counted, because they are most likely contributing some fat grams (such as cheese). Either way, you want to make sure you are counting them in to see how they help balance your meals or snacks and what effect it has on your blood sugar in certain amounts.

Dairy Products

	Cal.	Carbs (g)	Fat (g, %*)	Pro. (g)	Sat. (g)	Sod. (mg)
Milk (1 cup)						
Skim milk	90	13	0	9	0	130
Low-fat milk (1%)	120	14	2.5	11	1.5	160
Low-fat milk (2%)	130	13	5	10	3	140
Whole milk	150	13	8	8	5	125
Cottage cheese (1/2 cup)						
Low-fat cottage cheese	80	3	2 (22%)	13	1	340
Small curd	120	4	5 (38%)	14	3	410
Yogurt						
"Light" fat-free, flavored yogurts (6 ounces)	90	15	0	5	0	75
99% fat-free flavored yogurts (6 ounces)	170	33	2	5	1	80
Low-fat custard-style, flavored yogurt (6 ounces)	190	32	3	8	2	100

*Percent calories from fat

Cereal

Whether you prefer it hot, wet, or dry, most of us like some type of cereal. If you eat cereal at least three times a week, that means you sit down to a bowl of cereal about 156 times a year. So which cereals we choose to eat can make a big difference in, for one thing, the amount of fiber we get.

Most cereals these days are relatively low in fat, which is actually good because most cereal manufacturers use the partially hydrogenated type of vegetable oils. What distinguishes one cereal from another is usually its sugar and fiber content. I've listed the cereals with 4 grams (or more) of fiber per serving, starting with the highest-fiber cereals. The grams of carbohydrate for each are also listed in the table.

Many of you will probably do better with cereal as breakfast or as a snack, if you add some fat to this mostly carbohydrate meal. Low-fat milk is a pretty good way to do this (I've listed some milk in the table so you can count it in with your cereal totals). If you have room left in your carbohydrate breakfast budget, you can top your cereal with sliced banana or berries!

Cereal

	Cal.	Carb. (g)	Fat (g, %*)	Fib. (g)	Sod. (mg)
All-Bran Extra Fiber, 1/2 cup	50	20	1 (18%)	13	120
Fiber One, 1/2 cup	60	24	1 (15%)	13	130
All-Bran original, 1/2 cup	80	24	1 (11%)	10	65
100% Bran, 1/3 cup	80	22	.5 (6%)	8	120
Kellogg's Raisin Bran	200	47	1.5 (7%)	8	370
Post Raisin Bran	190	47	1 (5%)	8	300
Shredded Wheat 'n Bran, 1 1/4 cup	200	47	1 (4%)	8	0
Bite Size Frosted Mini-Wheats	200	48	1 (5%)	6	5
Cracklin Oat Bran, 3/4 cup	190	35	7 (33%)	6	170
Raisin Bran Crunch, 1 1/4 cup	210	50	1 (4%)	5	250
Total Raisin Bran	180	43	1 (5%)	5	240
Bran Flakes, 3/4 cup	100	24	.5 (4%)	5	220
Complete Wheat Bran Flakes, 3/4 cup	90	23	.5 (9%)	5	220
Crunchy Corn Bran, 3/4 cup	90	23	1 (10%)	5	250
Spoon Size Shredded Wheat	170	41	.5 (26%)	5	0
Mini-Wheats (Raisin), 3/4 cup	180	42	1 (5%)	5	5
Frosted Shredded Wheat	190	44	1 (5%)	5	10
100% Whole Grain Wheat Chex	180	41	1.5 (8%)	5	420
Fruit & Fibre (Dates, Raisins, and Walnuts)	210	42	3 (13%)	5	280
Grape Nuts, 1/2 cup	210	47	1 (4%)	5	350
Raisin Nut Bran, 3/4 cup	200	41	4 (18%)	5	250
Crisp-Raisin Oatmeal	210	45	2 (8%)	4	220
Banana Nut Crunch (Post)	250	43	6 (22%)	4	250
Great Grains 2/3 cup	200	40	4.5 (20%)	4	160
Crispy Wheats 'n' Raisins	190	45	1 (5%)	4	270
Healthy Choice Mueslix (2/3 cup)	200	41	3 (13%)	4	160
Toasted Oatmeal Squares (Quaker)	220	43	2.5 (12%)	4	260
Toasted Oatmeal (Quaker)	190	43	2 (9%)	4	65

*Percent calories from fat

If you're wondering where the Cheerios and whole-grain Wheaties are . . .

They contain 3 grams of fiber per serving so they didn't quite make the list. But just in case, the following chart lists the more popular cereals with 3 grams of fiber:

More cereal

	Cal.	Carb. (g)	Fat (g, %*)	Fib. (g)	Sod. (mg)
Cheerios	110	22	2 (16%)	3	280
Multi-Grain Cheerios Plus	110	24	1 (8%)	3	200
Whole Grain Wheaties	110	24	1 (8%)	3	220
Whole Grain Total	110	24	1 (8%)	3	200
Cranberry Almond Crunch	210	43	3 (13%)	3	200
Basic 4	200	43	3 (13%)	3	320
Grape Nuts Flakes, 3/4 cup	100	24	3 (13%)	3	140
Nutri-Grain Almond Raisin, 1 1/4 cup	180	38	2.5 (12%)	3	170

*Percent calories from fat

Crackers and cookies

Most manufacturers use hydrogenated vegetable oils to make their crackers and cookies, which means most of these products contribute those undesirable trans fatty acids. Until companies start using liquid canola oil to make their products, the only way to eat crackers and cookies that contain fewer trans fatty acids, then, is to choose crackers and cookies that are lower in fat overall. Look for the reduced-fat varieties of either—many taste terrific.

My family particularly likes the reduced-fat Hi Ho and Ritz crackers, reduced-fat Keebler Club Crackers, and the SnackWell's Wheat and Cracked Pepper crackers. If you like rye, there are fat-free rye crackers that you could try also.

Remember, you aren't supposed to eat half the box. Try and stick to a "serving" at a time. The amount of cookies and crackers per serving is listed on the box. In order to do this though, the crackers and cookies have to taste great and satisfy even the most hard-to-please palates. I've listed what I consider the better-tasting reduced fat cookies in the table below.

Cookies

	Cal.	Carbs. (g)	Fat (g, %*)
SnackWell's Double Chocolate Chip Cookies, 13	130	22	3 (21%)
SnackWell's Mint Creme, 2	110	19	3.5 (29%)
SnackWell's Creme Sandwich Cookies, 2	110	20	3 (25%)
Nabisco Reduced Fat Chips Ahoy! cookies, 3	140	22	5 (32%)
Nabisco Reduced Fat Oreo	130	25	3.5 (24%)
Nabisco Teddy Grahams Chocolatey Chip Cookies, 24	130	23	4.5 (31%)
Pepperidge Farm Reduced Fat Oatmeal Cookies, 1	100	18	3 (27%)

*Percent calories from fat
These cookies contain 1 to 2 g protein, less than or equal to 1 g fiber, about 1-1.5 g saturated fat, and 70-190 sodium per serving.

Convenient spaghetti sauces

In order to be included in the list of store-bought sauces that follows, the sauce had to contain canola or olive oil (our high monounsaturated fat oils). If you've tasted some of the bottled sauces before, I fully realize you may be rather skeptical about buying prepared sauces. This is different.

The marinara/spaghetti sauces are the only ones that sit on the shelf at room temperature—and they are really pretty good. You can always add in your own super-lean ground beef, mushrooms, garlic, onion, and other spices, if you want to dress them up a little. The rest of the sauces can be found either in the frozen food section (next to the frozen raviolis) or in the refrigerated "fresh pasta" section.

Pasta sauces

	Cal.	Carbs. (g)	Fat (g, %*)
Red Sauces (1/2 cup)			
Five Brothers			
Grilled Eggplant & Parmesan	100	13	3
Grilled Summer Vegetable	80	11	3
Mushroom & Garlic Grill	90	12	3
Marinara w/Burgundy Wine	90	11	3
Classico			
Tomato & Basil	50	9	1
Fire-Roasted Tomato & Garlic	60	10	1
Sutter Home			
Italian Style w/fresh onions and herbs	80	12	2
Basilla			
Roasted Garlic & Onion	80	12	3.5
Mushroom & Garlic	70	11	2
Tomato & Basil	70	12	1.5
Marinara	70	11	2
Pesto (1/4 cup)			
Contadino Reduced-Fat Pesto with Basil	230	111	8
Safeway Select Verdi Classic Pesto	240	72	2
Light Alfredo Sauce (1/4 cup)			
Contadina	80	5	5
Safeway Select Verdi	80	5	5

Most of the red sauces mentioned here contain 0.5 g or less saturated fat, 2 to 3 g protein, 2 to 3 g fiber, and between 390 and 610 mg sodium per serving. Most of the pesto or alfredo sauces contain 3 to 4 g protein, between 5 and 20 mg cholesterol, and about 500 mg or less sodium per serving.

For bottled spaghetti sauce (normally low in fat and high in carbohydrates), I've listed the brands that contain some olive or canola oil, which means they will contribute some monounsaturated fat. Some people may have better post-pasta blood sugars if there is some fat in there

High Monounsaturated Fat Salad Dressings and Spreads

	Cal.	Carbs. (g)	Fat (g)
Mayonnaise: 1 tablespoon*			
Safeway Select Real Mayonnaise w/canola	100	0	11
Spectrum Canola Mayo	100	0	12
Spectrum Lite Canola Eggless Mayonnaise	35	1	3
Salad dressing: 2 tablespoons**			
Kraft Special Collection			
Sun Dried Tomato	60	4	4.5
Italian Pesto	70	5	5.5
Balsamic Vinaigrette	110	1	12
Kraft—Light Done Right			
Red Wine Vinaigrette	50	3	4.5
Italian	50	2	4.5
Raspberry Vinaigrette	60	6	4
Cucumber Ranch	60	2	5.5
Catalina	80	9	5
Kraft			
Roasted Garlic Vinaigrette	50	3	4.5
Caesar Parmesan	60	1	5
Newman's Own			
Dynamite Lite Italian	45	3	4
Balsamic Vinaigrette	90	3	9
Bernstein's			
Italian Cheese and Garlic	110	2	11
Red Wine and Garlic Italian	110	2	11
Parmesan Garlic Ranch	140	2	14
Balsamic Italian	110	2	11

*Mayonnaise: 80 or less mg sodium and 1 g saturated fat per serving.
**Salad dressing: Between 230 and 480 mg sodium and 1 g saturated fat per serving.

somewhere. Obviously if you've found one you like that is fat-free, go for it. But if you haven't, give the ones on page 177 a try.

High monounsaturated fat salad dressings and spreads

The products on the previous page contain exclusively the high monounsaturated fat vegetable oils: canola oil, olive oil, or a combination of the two.

Sugar Products

Last but not least, here are a handful of sugar-free or reduced-sugar products that might help you cut down on some extra calories from carbohydrate.

Canned fruits in lightly sweetened juice offer fruits year-round with less sugar than regular canned fruits.

Half a cup of peaches canned in lightly sweetened peach juice contains 80 calories, 19 grams carbohydrate, 1 gram protein, 1 gram fiber, and 20 milligrams sodium.

Half a cup of apricot halves in lightly sweetened juice contains 60 calories, 16 grams carbohydrate, 0 grams fat, 0 grams protein, 1 gram fiber, and 10 milligrams sodium.

JELL-O sugar-free instant pudding is available in several flavors. One serving of chocolate contains 35 calories, 8 grams carbohydrate, 0 grams fat, < 1 gram protein, < 1 gram fiber, and 320 milligrams sodium.

JELL-O sugar-free gelatin desserts are available in several flavors. Use them in your favorite JELL-O recipes or as a quick, low-calorie snack.

Reduced-calorie pancake syrups can be found in regular and butter flavored. One-fourth of a cup contains about 100 calories, 25 grams carbohydrate, and 130 milligrams sodium.

Low-sugar and lite jelly and preserves come in all sorts of brands and flavors. Smucker's makes low-sugar jellies and preserves. A tablespoon contains 25 calories and 6 grams of carbohydrate.

Knott's Berry Farm makes light preserves. A tablespoon contains 20 calories and 5 grams of carbohydrate.

Chapter 7

Restaurant Rules to Eat By

Most people go to restaurants and try to steer clear of one thing—overtly high-fat, high-calorie menu selections. But people with diabetes often have a few more things they worry about when approaching the menu. You need to get a feel for how many carbohydrate grams you might be eating and whether it is something that tends to keep your after-meal blood sugars high or not. You might want to choose something that contributes a moderate amount of monounsaturated fat because many find this helps with blood sugar control. You might also be trying to keep saturated fat and trans fatty acids low and omega-3 fatty acids (found in fish and some plant foods) high, to help protect your heart. Many of you may also need to count protein and potassium if you are on dialysis.

That's quite a bit to have on your plate (so to speak.) All this could very well take the fun out of eating out, couldn't it? The trick is finding the happy medium between counting what you need to count and ordering and enjoying foods you like. It can be done. It takes a little practice. And having the grams of fat, fiber, and carbohydrate for various menu selections helps too.

If your doctor or dietitian has told you to limit sodium, some of the following choices are going to be better than others—some have much higher amounts of sodium. Watch the last column in the nutrition table on page 185-199 to see which ones those are.

Cutting fat and calories when eating out

Remember some people with diabetes control their blood sugar better if they aren't on a very low-fat diet but are on a moderate-fat diet (around 30 to 35 percent calories from fat). If you are in this group, it is particularly important that you choose monounsaturated fats and omega-3 and omega-9 fatty acids (olive oil, canola oil, fish) whenever possible. No matter which group you are in, though, you will want to avoid "high" animal fat foods that load on extra calories and saturated fat fast. One of the downfalls of eating out is the hefty portions of meat/dairy they often serve you. There are a few things you can do to keep this in check:

- The lean cuts of beef at restaurants are usually filet mignon, sirloin, sirloin tips, or chopped sirloin, while the fattier cuts are rib eye, prime rib, porterhouse, and T-bone.

- Make sure your "meat" dish is accompanied by lots of vegetables (beans when possible). The vegetables will help fill you up so you won't be tempted to overdo the meat, and the vegetables and beans help boost fiber totals too (good for your health and your blood sugars).

- Order the quarter-pounder instead of the third- or half-pound hamburger, and load up on lettuce, tomato, ketchup, and mustard, instead of mayonnaise, "special sauces," and cheese.

- Order the "petite" or "junior" portions of meat, prime rib, and steaks when available.
- Automatically cut your steak, pork chop, ham, or roasted chicken in half and take the rest home for tomorrow's sandwich.
- Ask the restaurant to make your "three-egg" omelet with Egg Beaters egg substitute or one egg blended with 3 egg whites.
- Avoid "extra cheese" and try to keep your servings of heavy cheese dishes (pizza, cheese enchiladas, lasagna, etc.) moderate.

To avoid excessive calories in general, you basically need to avoid ordering foods made with lots of:

- Butter or margarine: Each tablespoon of butter contains 11.5 grams fat and 102 calories.
- Mayonnaise: Each tablespoon of mayonnaise contains 11 grams of fat and 100 calories. Creamy mayonnaise-based salad dressings are dripping with fat grams. Remember one restaurant ladle adds up to two tablespoons of dressing worth around 25 grams of fat.
- Cream: One-quarter cup of liquid whipping cream contains 22 grams fat and 205 calories.
- Oil: Each tablespoon of oil contains 14 grams fat and 120 calories. Avoid deep fried anything, even if it is something healthful like chicken or seafood. Have it grilled instead.
- Sugar: It is loaded with calories. It's not that you can't have any. It helps to split the dessert you want to try with someone at the table or eat half and bring the other half home (if it isn't ice cream).

Restaurant chains menu picks

The steakhouse chain

There are many steakhouse chains across the country and most of them do **not** (shame on them) provide any nutrition information for their interested patrons. Hopefully it's obvious to avoid the gigantic, battered, and deep-fried onion, which, rumor has it, contains more than 100 grams of fat. Sampling, however, is manageable as long as it adds up to a few savored bites.

Even if you avoid everything that is deep-fried (not just because of the fat and calories but because anything deep-fried seems to cause high blood sugars for many people)—what about the other items? If you want to have steak, which ones are best for you? There are few things, no matter which steakhouse you're in, that will help put you in the nutritional driver's seat:

- Ask that the chef cook your meat without butter or added fat.
- Order your meat in small portions or have the kitchen cut a large portion in half and put the second half immediately into a doggy bag.
- Order your baked potato with butter and sour cream on the side.
- Order your salad with the dressing on the side.
- Trim the visible chunks of fat from your steak before you eat it.

I did some investigating and came up with the nutrition information for some typical steakhouse menu items. The actual nutrition content of your particular steakhouse item might be higher in fat and calories, but the following table will get you in the ballpark.

Menu Items: Steakhouses

	Carbs. (g)	Fat (g [%*])	Pro. (g)	Fib. (g)	Cals.
Entrées					
Grilled chicken	1	2 (15%)	25	n/a	120
Grilled chicken sandwich	39	4 (11%)	33	n/a	324
Grilled salmon (4 oz.)	1	10 (42%)	34	n/a	240
Sirloin tips w/peppers & onions	4	8 (35%)	27	n/a	203
Spicy BBQ chicken sandwich	45	5 (12%)	34	n/a	368
Homestyle chicken fillet	21	9 (37%)	13	n/a	217
Junior sirloin steak	0	10 (46%)	25	n/a	194
Filet mignon, 1 (5.5 oz. cooked)	0	15 (44%)	44	0	330
Smothered steak sandwich	36	15 (31%)	34	n/a	430
Sirloin steak	0	16 (51%)	34	n/a	285
Country steak with gravy	44	25 (42%)	32	n/a	530
Sides					
Baked potato, plain	31	0	3	3	130
Broccoli spears	5	0	3	3	35
Corn, 4 oz.	28	1.5 (9%)	4	3	120
BBQ beans (4 oz.)	25	2 (14%)	6	5	150
Rice pilaf (1/2 cup)	23	3.5 (23%)	2	.5	135
Dinner roll, 1	14	2 (22%)	2	1	85
Cornbread, 1 pc.	28	5 (26%)	4.5	1.5	175
Cinnamon apples	34	5 (26%)	0	2	172
Mashed potatoes, .5 cup	18	5 (35%)	2	2	115
Biscuit, 1	29	15 (50%)	5	1	270
Soups (1 cup)					
Vegetable beef	18	2 (15%)	7	3	120
Clam chowder, New England	17	9 (45%)	3	1.5	180
Chili w/beans	25	9 (30%)	23	5	270

*Percent calories from fat

Chili's

Chili's has a "Guiltless Grill" section in their menu, featuring about five lower-fat entrees ranging from 3 grams fat and 254 calories to 13 grams fat and 696 calories. All of these are really high in fiber too. To increase the fat grams a little (to an amount that encourages a better post-meal blood glucose) you can always have a side salad with some dressing or a few french fries. There are many other great choices on the Chili's menu too. The following selections have a good chance of fitting into your diabetic, carbo-counting eating plan.

Menu Items: Chili's

	Carbs. (g)	Fat (g [%*])	Fib. (g)	Cal.
Guiltless Grill				
Veggie pasta	98	11 (17%)	16	590
Veggie pasta with chicken	102	13 (17%)	17	696
Chicken platter	83	7 (11%)	12	563
Chicken sandwich	83	7 (12%)	18	527
Chicken salad with dressing	27	3 (11%)	6	254
Regular Menu				
Chicken caesar salad w/o dressing	29	21 (40%)	N/A	476
3 chicken tacos with rice and beans	137	33 (28 %)	N/A	1077
Cheesesteak (no fries)	61	35 (42%)	N/A	749
Chicken fajitas with toppings	75	47 (43%)	N/A	964
Turkey sandwich	55	34 (44%)	N/A	691

*Percent calories from fat

Denny's

Denny's should be commended for being one of the only restaurant chains that willingly offers nutrition information for every single menu item. I wish there were more restaurant chains like this one.

Menu Items: Denny's

	Carbs. (g)	Fat (g [%*])	Pro. (g)	Fib. (g)	Cal.	Sod. (mg)
Breakfast Menu						
Oatmeal	18	2 (18%)	5	3	100	175
Grits	18	0 (0%)	2	0	80	520
Egg Beater veggie omelette	29	N/A	N/A	4	N/A	N/A
French toast without syrup or butter	54	24 (42%)	16	3	507	594
Buttermilk hotcakes (3) without syrup or butter	95	7 (13%)	12	3	491	1,818
Ham, grilled slice	2	3 (29%)	15	0	94	761
Egg Beaters	1	5 (63%)	5	0	71	138
Toppings						
Maple-flavored syrup, 3 Tbs	36	0	0	0	143	26
Sugar-free syrup	9	0	0	0	23	71
Blueberry syrup	26	0	0	0	102	15
Whipped margarine	0	10	0	0	87	117
Cream cheese	1	10	2	0	100	90
Salads/Sandwiches/Soups						
Grilled Chicken Sandwich	52	19 (34%)	34	3	509	1,809
Garden Burger	75	33 (44%)	18	8	665	1,051
Charleston Chicken s/w	53	32 (45%)	35	4	632	1,967
Turkey breast w/ multigrain	39	26 (49%)	23	5	476	1,107
Garden Chicken Delite Salad	33	6 (18%)	30	6	300	1,300
Chili w/cheese topping	21	19 (42%)	26	7	401	1,039
Split pea soup	18	6 (37%)	8	2	146	819
Vegetable beef soup	11	1 (11%)	6	2	79	820
Chicken noodle	8	2 (30%)	2	0	60	640

Denny's (cont'd)

Dinners	Carbs. (g)	Fat (g [%*])	Pro. (g)	Fib. (g)	Cal.	Sod. (mg)
Pot Roast Dinner w/ gravy (add sides)	6	11 (37%)	40	0	265	1,165
Roast Turkey & Stuffing w/gravy (add sides)	63	27 (35%)	47	0	701	2,346
Grilled Chicken Breast Dinner (add sides)	0	4 (28%)	24	0	130	566
Grilled Alaskan Salmon Dinner (add sides)	1	4 (17%)	43	0	210	103
Chicken Strips (add sides)	55	25 (35%)	47	0	635	1,510
Side dishes						
Baked potato	43	0 (0%)	4	4	186	14
Vegetable rice pilaf	16	1 (11%)	2	1	85	325
Broccoli in butter sauce	7	2 (36%)	3	3	50	280
Corn in butter sauce	19	4 (30%)	3	5	120	260
Green peas in butter	14	2 (18%)	5	4	100	360
Carrots in honey glaze	12	3 (34%)	1	3	80	220
Desserts						
Low-fat choc chip yogurt	19	2 (16%)	4	1	110	60
"Shared" rootbeer/cola float	23	5 (32%)	1.5	0	140	54
"Shared" apple pie serving	30	10 (42%)	5	.5	215	195
"Shared" chocolate layer cake serving	21	6 (39%)	2	0	137	31
"Shared" cheesecake serving	24	13 (50%)	3	0	235	140

*Percent calories from fat

Menu Items: Boston Market

	Carbs. (g)	Fat (g [%*])	Pro. (g)	Fib. (g)	Cal.	Sod. (mg)
1/4 White Meat Chicken, no skin	2	4 (21%)	33	0	170	480
5 oz. Skinless Rotisserie Turkey Breast	1	1 (6%)	36	0	170	850
5 oz. (lean) Hearth Honey Ham	9	9 (38%)	30	0	210	1,490
Teriyaki Chicken 1/4 white w/skin	17	12 (32%)	40	0	340	890
Southwest Savory Chicken, 1 portion	26	15 (35%)	40	4	400	1,670
Baked Sweet Potato, 1	94	7 (15%)	6	10	460	510
BBQ Baked Beans, 3/4 cup	48	5 (17%)	8	12	270	540
Black Beans and Rice, 1 cup	45	10 (30%)	8	5	300	1,050
New Potatoes, 3/4 cup	25	2.5 (17%)	3	2	130	150
Red Beans and Rice, 1 cup	45	5 (19%)	8	4	260	1,050
Rice Pilaf, 2/3 cup	32	5 (25%)	5	2	180	600
Steamed Vegetables, (2/3 cup)	7	.5 (14%)	2	3	35	35
Zucchini Marinara, 3/4 cup	7	3 (41%)	1	2	60	330
Corn Bread, 1 mini loaf	33	6 (25%)	3	1	200	390
Turkey Sandwich, no cheese or sauce	61	3.5 (8%)	45	4	400	1,070
Ham Sandwich, no cheese or sauce	66	8 (16%)	25	4	440	1,450
Open-faced Turkey Sandwich	61	12 (22%)	37	4	500	2,170
BBQ Chicken Sandwich	84	9 (15%)	30	3	540	1,690
Chicken Noodle Soup, 1 cup	12	4.5 (31%)	11	2	130	1,310
Chicken Chili, 1 cup	21	7 (27%)	18	6	220	1,000

*Percent calories from fat

Menu Items: Olive Garden

	Carbs. (g)	Fat (g [%*])	Pro. (g)	Cal.	Sod. (mg)
Garden Fare lunch entrées					
Capellini Pomodoro	52	11 (28%)	9	340	700
Capellini Primavera	58	7 (19%)	14	350	820
Capellini Primavera with chicken	59	13 (23%)	39	510	1,550
Chicken Giardino	40	7 (21%)	20	300	910
Linguine alla Marinara	48	6 (20%)	8	280	510
Penne Arrabbiata	49	7 (22%)	8	300	530
Shrimp Primavera	53	9 (18%)	36	440	830
Garden Fare dinner entrées					
Capellini Pomodoro	84	17 (28%)	16	550	1,090
Capellini Primavera	99	12 (18%)	23	600	1,450
Capellini Primavera with chicken	101	18 (21%)	48	760	2,190
Chicken Giardino	59	8 (16%)	36	460	1,180
Grilled Chicken Capri	45	9 (17%)	58	500	640
Linguine alla Marinara	79	9 (19%)	14	450	770
Penne Arrabbiata	67	11 (23%)	12	410	800
Shrimp Primavera	103	14 (15%)	69	830	1,390
Other					
Minestrone Soup (6 oz)	18	1 (9%)	5	100	610
Plain Breadstick	26	1.5 (10%)	5	140	270

*Percent calories from fat
Fiber information was not available for these items.

Good choices at pizza parlors

Some pizza chains have higher-fat pizza crust, while others have the more traditional, bread-type crust. I trust you can tell the difference. But in case you can't, lay your slice of pizza on a thick napkin. Do the grease spots form a triangle where the crust was? The grease from the crust is an indication of its fat content. It's best to frequent the pizza places that have the more traditional bread crusts—that's half the battle. Domino's, for example, makes a hand tossed pizza crust and a pan crust. The hand tossed is the one you want to ask for, because it has half the fat and saturated fat of deep-dish pizza.

The second factor in choosing the healthier pizza pie is the toppings—the cheese and all the trimmings. If you ask them to make the pizza with less cheese, this will definitely help. I know you feel silly doing this, but many of these restaurants really do put on more cheese than pizza really needs. If you are used to the typical combination pizza (sausage and pepperoni), this next tip could be a tough one. If you top your pizza with items that don't add fat calories, but instead add nutrition and fiber—you are hitting the nutrition jackpot. You see, people usually don't have any vegetables with their pizza meal (unless they order a salad), so why not top your pizza with the vegetables you like and make it a more complete meal? Hopefully you like a couple of the following vegetable toppings: peppers, onions, mushrooms, zucchini, fresh tomatoes, broccoli, artichoke hearts, and also fruits such as pineapple. The leaner meat toppings are Canadian bacon and ham.

Blood sugar beware . . .

Pizza seems to be one of those foods that raises blood sugar beyond what the grams of carbohydrate could explain. You might find you tolerate your pizza better if you have a side salad, heavy on the kidney beans, before you eat your pizza. This is probably not a good time to be eating a big slice of cake either. Try two large-size slices of cheese pizza and see how your blood sugar fares. Two slices will bring you to about 45 g of carbohydrate, 10 g of fat, 13 g of protein, 317 calories, and 669 mg sodium. Two deep-dish slices bring you to 54 g of carbohydrate, 20 g of fat, 18 g of protein, 455 calories, and 1,030 mg of sodium.

Good choices at sandwich shops

There are really great sandwich choices at the following sandwich restaurants. They are great places to go when you have a few minutes and/or a few dollars for lunch. The nutrition facts for the sandwiches are analyzed using white bread. If you opt for the whole- or part-wheat selections, your grams of fiber might go up about 2 to 4 grams per sandwich.

Menu Items: Blimpie (per 6-inch sub)

	Carbs. (g)	Fat (g [%*])	Pro. (g)	Fib. (g)	Cal.	Sod. (mg)
Blimpie Best	47	13 (28%)	26	4	410	1,480
Ham and Swiss	47	13 (27%)	25	5	430	970
Turkey	51	4.5 (13%)	19	3	320	690
Roast Beef	47	4.5 (12%)	27	2	340	870
Club	53	13 (26%)	30	3	450	1,350
Grilled Chicken	52	9 (20%)	28	2	400	960
Grilled Chicken Salad	13	12 (31%)	47	0	350	1,190

*Percent of calories from fat

Subway

Unless noted, the following nutrition data does not include cheese and condiments, such as mayonnaise and salad dressing. If you add mayonnaise or salad dressing, you'll need to add this into the equation (see table below). Good news though, Subway offers light mayonnaise. Other condiments available upon request are mustard, vinegar, and an olive oil blend.

Menu Items: Subway

	Carbs. (g)	Fat (g [%*])	Pro (g)	Cal.	Sod. (mg)
Per 6-inch Subs					
Veggie Delite	44	3 (11%)	9	237	593
Turkey Breast	46	4 (12%)	18	289	1,403
Turkey Breast & Ham	46	5 (15%)	18	295	1,361
Ham	45	5 (15%)	19	302	1,319
Roast Beef	45	5 (15%)	20	303	939
Subway Club	46	5 (14%)	21	312	1,352
Seafood & Crab (made w/lite mayo)	45	10 (26%)	20	347	884
Roasted Chicken Breast	47	6 (16%)	27	348	978
Steak & Cheese	47	10 (23%)	30	398	1,117
Subway Melt (includes cheese)	46	12 (28%)	23	382	1,746
Deli-Style Sandwiches (on deli style roll)					
Turkey	38	4 (15%)	12	235	944
Ham	37	4 (15%)	11	234	773
Roast Beef	38	4 (15%)	13	245	638
Tuna (w/lite mayo)	38	9 (29%)	11	279	583
Salads (not including dressing)					
Veggie Delite	10	1 (18%)	2	51	308
Turkey Breast	12	2 (18%)	11	102	1,117
Subway Club	12	3 (21%)	11	126	1,067
Roast Beef	11	3 (23%)	12	117	654
Ham	11	3 (23%)	12	116	1,034
Turkey Breast & Ham	11	3 (25%)	11	109	1,076
Roasted Chicken Breast	13	4 (22%)	20	162	693
Steak & Cheese	13	8 (34%)	22	212	832

*Percent calories from fat

Good choices at fast food chains

It's too easy to eat a horrendously high-fat, high-calorie meal at your average fast food chain. But probably the biggest problems are they are the more heart-damaging types of fat, and you'd be hard pressed to find a fruit or vegetable to munch on. Some of the restaurants now offer side salads and fat-free or light salad dressing to go with your sandwich selection. If you know you will be eating a fast food, bring along some fruit and raw vegetables (carrots, celery) to help round off the meal. I know this sounds totally impractical. But if you eat fast food often, this is an important habit to get into.

Menu Items: Burger King

	Carbs. (g)	Fat (g [%*])	Pro. (g)	Fib. (g)	Cal.	Sod. (mg)
Whopper Jr. (without mayo)	28	15 (44%)	19	2	320	530
Hamburger	27	15 (44%)	19	1	320	520
BK Big Fish sandwich (no tartar sauce)	59	14 (27%)	23	3	460	850
BK Broiler Chicken sandwich (no mayo)	45	9 (22%)	29	2	370	1,060
Chicken sandwich (without mayo)	54	20 (36%)	26	2	500	1,400
Chick'N Crisp (without mayo)	37	16 (39%)	16	3	360	890
Small Vanilla Shake	56	7 (19%)	10	1	330	250
Small French Fries	32	13 (32%)	2	2	250	550

*Percent calories from fat

When it comes to burgers, bigger is not better. The smaller the hamburger, the lower the percent of calories from fat. Some of this has to do with the smaller hamburgers having more bun per square inch of burger. But some of it has to do with the bigger burgers getting the fancier (and higher fat) sauces while the small burgers are served with ketchup and mustard. Each fast food chain has its pluses and minuses. Take a look at the list below to find some selections you would enjoy in each.

Menu Items: Carl's Jr.

	Carbs. (g)	Fat (g [%*])	Pro. (g)	Fib. (g)	Cal.	Sod. (mg)
Charbroiled BBQ sandwhich	37	3 (10%)	25	2	280	830
Char. Chicken Salad-To-Go (fat-free dressing)	16	7 (29%)	25	3	215	1,210
Jr. Hamburger	34	13 (35%)	18	1	330	480
Sour cream and chives potato	70	14 (29%)	7	6	430	135
Charbroiled Santa Fe Chicken sandwich	32	31 (55%)	28	2	510	1,240
Charbroiled Sirloin Steak sandwich	50	26 (38%)	33	2	580	110
Carl's Catch Fish sandwich	50	27 (48%)	18	1	510	1030
French Fries	37	14 (43%)	5	3	290	170
Bran Raisin Muffin	61	13 (32%)	7	6	370	410

*Percent calories from fat

Menu Items: Jack in the Box

	Carbs. (g)	Fat (g [%*])	Pro. (g)	Fib. (g)	Cal.	Sod. (mg)
Chicken Teriyaki Bowl	128	4 (5%)	26	3	670	1,730
Pancakes with Bacon	59	9 (22%)	12	3	370	1,020
Chicken Fajita Pita	25	9 (29%)	24	3	280	840
Breakfast Jack	30	12 (39%)	17	1	280	920
Hamburger	30	12 (38%)	12	2	280	560
Hamburger with Cheese	30	16 (45%)	14	2	320	760
Chicken Breast Pieces (5)	24	17 (42%)	27	1	360	970
Garden Chicken Salad	8	9 (40%)	23	3	200	420
Side Salad	3	3 (54%)	2	3	50	75
Low Calorie Italian Dressing (4 tbsp)	2	1.5 (54%)	0	0	25	670

*Percent calories from fat

Menu Items: McDonald's

	Carbs. (g)	Fat (g [%*])	Pro. (g)	Fib. (g)	Cal.	Sod. (mg)
Hamburger	34	9 (31%)	13	2	250	580
Cheeseburger	35	13 (37%)	15	2	320	820
Grilled Chicken Deluxe	38	20 (41%)	27	4	440	1,040
Grilled Chicken Deluxe (no mayo)	38	5 (15%)	27	4	300	930
Grilled Chicken Salad Deluxe w/1 pkg. fat-free Herb dressing	18	1.5 (8%)	21	3	170	570
Grilled Chicken Salad with 1/2 packet Caesar Dressing	10.5	8.5 (38%)	22	3	200	465
Egg McMuffin	27	12 (38%)	17	1	290	790
Hotcakes (plain)	58	9 (23%)	9	2	340	540
Hotcakes w/2 pats margarine & syrup	18	(26%)	9	2	610	600
Low-fat Apple Bran Muffin	61	3 (10%)	6	3	300	380
Vanilla Reduced Fat Ice Cream Cone	23	4.5 (27%)	4	0	150	75
Small Shake (all flavors)	60	9 (22%)	11	0	360	180

*Percent calories from fat
**The carbohydrate and calorie count would reduce if only 1/2 syrup packet was used.

Menu Items: Kentucky Fried Chicken

	Carbs.	Fat (g [%*])	Pro. (g)	Fiber (g)	Cal.	Sod. (mg)
Tender Roast Chicken Breast w/out skin	1	4.3 (23%)	31.4	0	169	797
Tender Roast Chicken Thigh w/o skin	< 1	5.5 (46%)	13	0	106	312
BBQ Flavored Chicken sandwich	28	8 (28%)	17	2	256	782
BBQ Baked Beans	33	3 (14%)	6	6	190	760
Corn on the Cob	35	1.5 (9%)	5	2	150	20
Green Beans	7	1.5 (30%)	1	3	45	730
Mean Greens	11	3 (38%)	4	5	70	650

*Percent calories from fat

Menu Items: Wendy's

	Carbs. (g)	Fat (g [%*])	Pro. (g)	Fib. (g)	Cal.	Sod. (mg)
Sandwiches						
Grilled Chicken	35	8 (23%)	27	2	310	790
Jr. Hamburger	34	10 (33%)	15	2	270	610
Jr. Cheeseburger	34	13 (36%)	17	2	320	830
Spicy Chicken	43	15 (33%)	28	2	410	1,280
Plain Single	31	16 (40%)	24	2	360	580
Breaded Chicken	44	18 (37%)	28	2	440	840
Pitas·						
Garden Veggie	52	17 (38%)	11	5	400	760
Chicken Caesar	48	18 (33%)	34	4	490	1,320
Garden Ranch Chicken	51	18 (34%)	30	5	480	1,180
Salads··						
Side Salad	5	3 (45%)	4	2	60	180
Caesar Side Salad	7	5 (41%)	10	1	110	650
Deluxe Garden	9	6 (49%)	7	3	110	350
Grilled Chicken	9	8 (36%)	25	3	200	720
Dressing (2 tablespoons)						
Italian, reduced-fat	2	3			40	340
Ranch, reduced-fat	2	5			60	240
French, fat-free	8	0			35	150
Other						
Sour Cream & Chives Potato	74	6 (14%)	8	8	380	40
Broccoli & Cheese Potato	80	14 (27%)	9	9	470	470
Chili, small serving	2	17 (30%)	15	5	210	800

·The pitas are made with reduced-fat caesar vinaigrette (70 calories, 7 grams fat per tablespoon) or a reduced-fat garden ranch sauce (50 calories, 4.5 grams fat per tablespoon).

··The salad values below do not include salad dressing. Add in the nutrition info for the salad dressing of your choice.

+Order these sandwiches with ketchup or reduced-calorie honey mustard instead of the mayonnaise and you'll reduce the sandwich totals by about 3 grams fat for ketchup and 1.5 grams fat for the honey mustard.

* Percent calories from fat

Bagel shops

I love fresh bagels! Spread with light cream cheese, they are one of my favorite breakfasts. Bagels look innocent enough but they can be trouble for some people with diabetes. There's something about those 40-ish grams of carbohydrates that seems to make normal blood sugars difficult first thing in the morning for many people with type II diabetes. But there are a few things you can do to try to improve your post-bagel blood sugars.

Try whole-grain bagels or oat-bran bagels to see if that makes a difference. And make sure you balance your mostly carbohydrate bagel with some protein and a little fat. You can do this by spreading your bagel with light cream cheese or filling a savory bagel with some reduced-fat cheese and a slice of lean ham. Here is what some of these options add up to:

Menu Items: Bagel Shop

	Carbs. (g)	Fat (g [%*])	Pro. (g)	Fib. (g)	Cal.	Sod. (mg)
Bagel	38	6 (22%)	10	1.5	254	507
Whole-Grain Bagel	33	5.5 (23%)	9	3.5	212	414

*Percent calories from fat
Note: All listings include 1/8 cup light cream cheese.

Donut/Coffee shop chain

Here is the nutrition information from a national donut/coffee shop chain. We all find ourselves in these places every now and then, and we all probably crave donuts every once in a while. When we do—here is some of the nutrition information that can help you make your choices.

Menu Items: Donut/Coffee Shops

	Carbs. (g)	Fat (g [%*])	Pro. (g)	Fib. (g)	Cal.	Sod. (mg)
French cruller	24	7.5 (40%)	1	2	170	140
Cake donut, glazed	23	10 (47%)	3	2	192	180
Cinnamon bun	31	10 (39%)	4	6	220	190
Jelly donut	25	12 (48%)	4	3	221	190
Croissant	26	12 (47%)	5	7	231	424
Yeast donut	26	14 (50%)	4	3	242	205
Fruit danish	45	16 (42%)	5	3	335	333
Cheese danish	29	25 (62%)	6	5	350	319

*Percent calories from fat

Chapter 8

Smart Snacking

D o the words chips, cookies, ice cream, candy bars, or crackers mean anything to you? These higher-calorie, fat, or sugar foods represent our more popular snack foods. But to start snacking wisely, you don't necessarily need to trade all your Chips Ahoy cookies for carrot sticks, or your carton of ice cream for a carton of tofu. We can make smarter snack choices by choosing foods that are higher in fiber and important nutrients, feature carbohydrates with lower glycemic indexes, and that are balanced with some protein and some of the more heart helpful fats such as monounsaturated fats and omega-3 fatty acids.

Do you feel guilty when you get a snack attack? You are not alone. Snacking has gotten a bad rap in the past, mainly because of the types of foods we tend to snack on. But really, eating smaller, more frequent meals and snacks can be particularly helpful for people with diabetes. Small meals/snacks eaten every 2 1/2 to 3 hours tend to translate into more stable blood sugars throughout the day.

Some people with diabetes need to eat snacks to help prevent low blood glucose levels. These healthful snacks can be eaten before going to bed, exercising, or at other times when hypoglycemia tends to strike. For the people with diabetes who are more at risk of having high blood sugars (hyperglycemia), smart snacks would include higher-fiber, lower-glycemic index ingredients.

Soluble fiber snacks

Foods rich in soluble fiber make for great snacks because soluble fiber leaves the stomach slowly, encouraging better blood sugars and making you feel satisfied longer. Here are some possible snack ingredients that are high in soluble fiber:

- Peas and beans.
- Oats and oat bran.
- Barley.
- Some fruits (apples, peaches, citrus, mango, plums, kiwi, pears, berries).
- Some vegetables (artichokes, celery root, sweet potatoes, parsnips, turnips, acorn squash, brussels sprouts, cabbage, green peas, broccoli, carrots, cauliflower, asparagus, beets).

TIP #1. Whole-grain snacks are a step in the right direction.

The latest research suggests that people who eat whole grains have the lowest incidence of diabetes. They appear to increase the efficiency of insulin so that less is required to metabolize the sugar.

Adding other plant foods that contribute some fat and/or protein into our snack recipes, such as nuts, soy foods, olive and canola oil, and avocado, may also help minimize high blood sugars resulting from traditionally high-carbohydrate snacks.

I've collected the following snack recipes, keeping all these tips in mind, to help you practice smarter snacking and encourage better blood sugars:

10 Smart snack recipes

 ## Strawberry Lemonade Smoothie

Makes 1 smoothie.

- 1 cup frozen (unsweetened) whole strawberries or 3/4 cup sliced
- 1/2 cup prepared sugar-free lemonade (such as Crystal Lite)
- 1/2 cup low-fat lemon, vanilla, or plain yogurt

1. Add all ingredients to blender or food processor and puree until well blended (about 1 minute).

2. Pour into a serving cup and add a straw!

Per serving: 165 calories, 6 g protein, 32 g carbohydrate, 1.8 g fat, .8 g saturated fat, 5 mg cholesterol, 2.2 g fiber, 73 mg sodium. Calories from fat: 10 percent. Plus 87 mg vitamin C, and—210 mg calcium!

After speaking with a few bagel-lovers, I thought I would calculate how to make a better bagel snack. Bagels are mostly carbohydrates, so it is important to top them with something that will add some protein and fat into the snack equation . . . this will make the bagel more satisfying and the energy will hit the bloodstream more slowly and last longer. This topping could be a little bit of peanut butter, some light cream cheese, or a slice of reduced-fat cheese and a slice of turkey breast.

The other key to a better bagel snack is eating whole wheat or whole grain if possible. This will pump some fiber into the picture and whole grains also contribute vitamin and minerals and phytochemicals that you aren't getting in bagels made with refined flour.

 TIP #2. Some foods do not cause high blood sugar.

Even in large amounts and if eaten alone, the following foods are not likely to result in a substantial rise in blood sugar:

- Meat.
- Poultry.
- Fish.

- Avocados.
- Salad vegetables.
- Cheese.
- Eggs.

[Am J Clin Nutr 2002;76:5-56, Foster-Powell et al., International table of glycemic index and glycemic load values: 2002]

Bagel and Cream Cheese

Makes 1 bagel snack.

- 1/2 whole-wheat or whole-grain bagel, toasted or untoasted
- 1 Tbs. of light cream cheese

Per serving: 108 calories, 2.7 g fiber, 4.5 g protein, 16.5 g carbohydrate, 2.9 g fat, 1.8 g saturated fat, 7.5 mg cholesterol, 210 mg sodium. Calories from fat: 24 percent.

Peanut Butter Banana Fana

Makes 2 snack servings.

- 1 banana
- 2 Tbs. smooth peanut butter (reduced-fat can also be used)
- Topping to roll banana in, such as cake-decorating sprinkles, or Rice Krispies cereal.

1. Peel banana. Place on piece of foil and freeze for 1 hour. Meanwhile remove peanut butter from refrigerator and bring to room temperature (so it's more spreadable).

2. Using a dinner knife, spread 2 Tbs. of the peanut butter all around the banana.

3. Roll in food topping of choice (such as 1/2 cup of Rice Krispies cereal, etc . . .)

4. Place on foil sheet and refrigerate for 1 hour. It's ready to eat!

Per serving (with Rice Krispies cereal): 175 calories, 5.5 g protein, 22 g carbohydrate, 8 g fat, 1 g saturated fat, 0 mg cholesterol, 2.4 g fiber, 55 mg sodium. Calories from fat: 42 percent.

 TIP #3. Low glycemic index foods are less refined.

Low glycemic index foods are generally less refined than their higher glycemic index counterparts. For example, white bread has a glycemic index of 105 and a glycemic load (glycemic index multiplied by the dietary carbohydrate content) of 10, while Healthy Choice Hearty 7 Grain bread has a glycemic index of 79 and a glycemic load of 8. Corn flakes has a glycemic index of 130 and a glycemic load of 24, while Raisin Bran cereal has a glycemic index of 87 (plus or minus 7) and a glycemic load of 12.

 ## Quick Vegetable Bean Salad

One serving of this quick salad gives you a dose of alpha and beta carotene, folic acid, vitamin C, fiber (and plant omega-3 fatty acids from the canola oil). If you want to make this more of a meal, stir in a can of albacore tuna to add fish omega-3 fatty acids and some protein into the picture.
Makes 8 servings.

- 3 cups baby carrots, diced or thinly sliced carrots
- 3 cups broccoli florets cut into bite-sized pieces
- 1 15-ounce can kidney beans, rinsed and drained well

- 1/2 cup finely chopped mild onion (use less if desired).
- 1/2 cup "1/3 less fat" bottled vinaigrette made with canola or olive oil. (I use Seven Seas 1/3 less fat Red Wine Vinaigrette with canola.)
- 1 6-oz. can albacore tuna in water (optional).

1. Combine carrot pieces with 1/4 cup water in a microwave-safe covered dish and cook on high about 3 to 5 minutes (or until just barely tender). Drain well and add to medium-sized serving bowl.

2. Combine broccoli pieces with 1/4 cup water in a microwave-safe covered dish and cook on high about 3 to 5 minutes (or until just barely tender). Drain well and add to medium-sized serving bowl.

3. Add beans, chopped onion, and vinaigrette (and tuna if desired) to serving bowl. Toss well to blend.

Per serving: 110 calories, 5 g protein, 19 g carbohydrate, 2.5 g fat, 0 g saturated fat, 0 mg cholesterol, 7 g fiber, 310 mg sodium. Calories from fat: 20 percent.

TIP #4. Go ahead get nutty.

An ounce of most nuts will add about 170 calories (with around 7 grams carbohydrate, 6 grams protein, and 15 grams fat). Which nuts are best? Hazelnuts and almonds are lowest in saturated fat, with macadamia and hazelnuts being the highest in monounsaturated fat (this is a good thing). Pistachios and macadamia nuts were highest in fiber (about 3 grams per ounce) with walnuts scoring highest in omega-3 fatty acids.

Yogurt Parfait

Yogurt makes a great snack, but day after day it can get a bit boring . . . one way to make it a little more interesting is to make a parfait with layers of yogurt, fresh fruit and low-fat granola. Here's one way to do this.

Makes 1 parfait.

Layer the following in a parfait glass: (repeat layers)

- 1/8 cup fresh fruit (such as berries or sliced peaches)
- 1/8 cup low-fat or regular yogurt (flavor of your choice)
- 1/8 cup low-fat granola

Per parfait: 160 calories, 5 g protein, 32 g carbohydrate, 2.5 g fat, .4 g saturated fat, 3 mg cholesterol, 2.6 g fiber, 80 mg sodium. Calories from fat: 12 percent. Plus 96 mg calcium.

Chilled melon is a refreshing afternoon or evening snack. Make a bowl of melon cubes or balls, cover the bowl, and keep it in the refrigerator for a quick snack.

 TIP #5. Yodel for yogurt.

A container of light fruit yogurt (low-fat and with artificial sweeteners) is a great snack at school or on the go. A 7-ounce container has about 13 grams of available carbohydrates and a glycemic index of 20, adding up to a glycemic load of only 2! Even the regular fruit yogurts (with added sugar) have about 31 grams of available carbohydrate (per 7 ounces) and a glycemic index of 47, adding up to a glycemic load of 10.

Melon Medley

Makes 4 snack servings.

- 3 cups honeydew melon balls or cubes
- 3 cups cantaloupe balls or cubes

In serving bowl, toss melon to mix.

Per serving: 87 calories, 1.6 g protein, 21.8 g carbohydrates, .5 g fat, 0 g saturated fat, 0 mg cholesterol, 1.7 g fiber, 23 mg sodium. Calories from fat: 4 percent

 ## Pear and Jarlsberg Lite

This is one of my favorite snacks . . . pairing pear wedges with a nicely flavored cheese such as Jarlsberg Lite or Gruyere. What a great way to work another fruit serving into my day!

Per serving (1 sliced pear with 1 ounce of sliced Jarlsberg Lite): 202 calories, 9 grams protein, 32.5 g carbohydrate, 5.5 g fat (3 g saturated fat, 1.6 g monounsaturated fat, .3 g polyunsaturated fat), 15 mg cholesterol, 5 g fiber, 150 mg sodium, Calories from fat: 24 percent

 ## Mini Turkey Melts

This is a snack I make for my daughter and myself often. It works well with the toaster oven.

Makes 2 snack servings.

- 10 Triscuits
- 5 thin slices of turkey breast (we like peppered turkey breast), cut in half
- 2 oz. shredded, reduced-fat cheese of choice (Jarlsberg Lite, cheddar, jack)

1.   Place 10 Triscuits in a toaster oven pan. Top each with half a slice of turkey (fold it over to fit).

2.   Top the turkey with shredded cheese.

3.   Broil in toaster oven, watching carefully, until cheese is nicely melted.

Per serving: 214 calories, 21 g protein, 16 g carbohydrate, 7 g fat (3.5 g saturated fat, 2.2 g monounsaturated fat, .1 g polyunsaturated fat), 40 mg cholesterol, 2 g fiber, 260 mg sodium (not including the sodium from the turkey—the sodium in turkey slices varies greatly by brand). Calories from fat: 29 percent.

"Healthy Pop" Jolly Time Popcorn

You knew it was coming. Sooner or later I would have to list microwave popcorn as a snack! The microwave popcorn companies usually use partially hydrogenated oils in their products, so you can bet many of the fat grams listed per serving are trans fatty acids. The lower-fat the popcorn, the lower the amount of trans fatty acids!

All you need is a popcorn packet and a microwave—at home or at school or even at the swim club—you are good to go.

There are a few brands with a 94-percent fat free (or thereabouts) microwave popping corn. I'm going to give you the nutritional analysis for Jolly Time's Healthy Pop Butter Flavor Microwave Pop Corn—mainly because it's the type my daughters seem to like.

Per serving (5 cups popped—about 2 1/2 servings per bag): 90 calories, 2 grams fat, 2 grams saturated fat, 0 mg cholesterol, 210 mg sodium, 23 grams carb, 9 grams dietary fiber, and 4 grams protein.

Wendy's Side Salad

I found myself in the Wendy's drive-through recently ordering side salads for my girls and me as we were rushing to the orthodontist and all in need of an afternoon snack. It's actually a fresh and colorful salad and, best of all, it's on the 99-cents menu!

Per serving: (side salad and dressed with half of a packet (2.5 ounces total) of reduced-fat creamy ranch dressing): 90 calories, 10.5 g carbohydrate, 2.5 g protein, 4.5 g fat, .7 g saturated fat, 7 mg cholesterol, about 2.5 g fiber, and 325 mg sodium.

TIP #6. Portable fruit.

Fruit can travel well in your backpack and comes in handy for a quick pick-me-up. Many fruits offer just enough carbohydrates with a nice dose of fiber. The following fruits have a low glycemic load (5 or less per serving):

- Cherries, glycemic load of 3 per (4 1/4 ounce) serving.
- Grapefruit, glycemic load of 3 per (4 1/4 ounce) serving.
- Kiwifruit, glycemic load of 5 per (4 1/4 ounce) serving.
- Oranges, glycemic load of 5 per (4 1/4 ounce) serving.
- Peaches (fresh or canned in juice), glycemic load of 4 per (4 1/4 ounce) serving.
- Pears, glycemic load of 4 per (4 1/4 ounce) serving.
- Plums, glycemic load of 3 per (4 1/4 ounce) serving.
- Cantaloupe, glycemic load of 4 per (4 1/4 ounce) serving.
- Strawberries, glycemic load of 1 per (4 1/4 ounce) serving.

Conclusion

You've heard the expression "you can lead a horse to water but you can't make him drink." I have been dragging my type II father (whom I love with all my heart) to the water for 15 years, and . . . well, he's not drinking. Oh sure, every now and then he might sip the water a little, or dip his toe in it, but he's not drinking. He just hasn't been interested in controlling his blood sugars. He won't write down what he is eating and the resultant blood sugars so that we can figure out patterns.

For 15 years I have watched him slowly lose his ability to drive, walk, travel. We are at the point where every month he is in the hospital for congestive heart or leg infections. Even now he isn't interested in controlling his blood sugars. All I can do now is just love him, keep him company when my mom is working a long day, scratch his back (one of his favorite things), and just generally savor every precious moment my children and I get to spend with him.

I applaud you for being motivated enough to improve your health and diabetes that you finished this book. I can't say I know exactly what you're going through, because I don't personally have type II diabetes...yet. But I do understand. And if this book has somehow made your life with diabetes more enjoyable and more comfortable, than all the long hours of writing and research were well worth it.

Glossary

atherosclerosis Disease involving clogging, narrowing, and hardening of the body's arteries and blood vessels.

carbohydrate Compound contained in dietary sugars and starches.

cardiovascular Related to the heart and blood vessels.

dialysis Process used to filter waste products from blood in patients whose kidneys are not able to do this.

diverticulosis Potentially dangerous condition in which the colon develops numerous small sacs or pouches.

epidemic Affecting a large portion of a population.

etiology Cause or origin, specifically of a disease.

excrete To discharge or eliminate from the body.

glucose Form of carbohydrate (sugar) processed by the body. People with diabetes often need to monitor the level of glucose in their blood.

glycemic index Ranking of foods based on their effect on the body's blood-glucose levels.

hypertension High blood pressure.

insulin Protein produced by the pancreas that aids in the metabolism of carbohydrates.

metabolism Body process involving the assimilation of food and the production of energy and waste products.

myocardial infarction Heart attack caused by a blockage in the flow of blood to the heart.

obesity Condition of having excessive body fat.

omega-3 fatty acids Potentially helpful dietary components found in abundance in fish and green leafy vegetables.

pancreas Large gland that secretes insulin and digestive enzymes.

pharmacological Related to medicinal or therapeutic drugs.

phytochemicals Chemicals related to plants.

sedentary Not active.

serum Watery portion of blood.

soluble Capable of being dissolved.

systolic Related to the contraction, or pumping, of the heart.

For More Information

American Diabetes Association
1701 North Beauregard Street
Alexandria, VA 22311
800-DIABETES (800-342-2383)
Web site: http://www.diabetes.org
Founded in 1940, the American Diabetes Association is the United States' leading nonprofit health organization providing diabetes research, information, and advocacy.

Children with Diabetes Foundation
685 E. Wiggins Street
Superior, CO 80027
(303) 475-4312
Web site: http://www.cwdfoundation.org
E-mail: info@CWDFoundation.org
The Children with Diabetes Foundation aims to assist young people living with diabetes and support the work of scientists and physicians throughout the world searching for a cure.

National Diabetes Information Clearinghouse
1 Information Way
Bethesda, MD 20892-3560
(800) 860–8747
Web site: http://diabetes.niddk.nih.gov
E-mail: ndic@info.niddk.nih.gov
The National Diabetes Information Clearinghouse (NDIC) collects and disseminates information about diabetes. The NDIC is a service of the National Institute of Diabetes and Digestive and Kidney Diseases (NIDDK), part of the National Institutes of Health (NIH), which is part of the U.S. Department of Health and Human Services.

Web Sites

Due to the changing nature of Internet links, Rosen Publishing has developed an online list of Web sites related to the subject of this book. This site is updated regularly. Please use this link to access the list:

http://www.rosenlinks.com/tmwe/diab

For Further Reading

American Diabetes Association. *American Diabetes Association Complete Guide to Diabetes*. New York, NY: Bantam Dell, 2006.

Becker, Gretchen. *The First Year: Type 2 Diabetes: An Essential Guide for the Newly Diagnosed*. Emeryville, CA: Marlowe & Company, 2006.

Grunes, Barbara. *Diabetes Snacks, Treats, and Easy Eats: 130 Recipes You'll Make Again and Again*. Chicago, IL: Surrey Books, 2003.

Loy, Bo Nasmyth, and Spike Nasmyth Loy. *487 Really Cool Tips for Kids with Diabetes*. Alexandria, VA: ADA Publishing, 2004.

Loy, Bo Nasmyth, and Spike Nasmyth Loy. *Getting a Grip on Diabetes*. Alexandria, VA: ADA Publishing, 2007.

Moran, Katherine J. *Diabetes: The Ultimate Teen Guide* (It Happened to Me). Lanham, MD: Scarecrow Press, 2006.

Rubin, Alan L. *Diabetes for Dummies*. New York, NY: Wiley and Sons, 2004.

Warshaw, Hope. *American Diabetes Association Guide to Healthy Fast Food Eating*. Alexandria, VA: ADA Publishing, 2006.

Warshaw, Hope S., and Karmeen Kulkarni. *ADA Complete Guide to Carb Counting*. Alexandria, VA: ADA Publishing, 2004.

Index

A

A-arachidonic acid, 58
allacin, 62, 66
almonds, food tips on, 58
alpha-linolenic acid, 89, 107
alphalipoic acid as antioxidant, 106
American Association of Certified Diabetes Educators, The, 16
American Diabetes Association, 16
American Dietetic Association's National Center for Nutrition and Dietetics, The, 16
American Heart Association, 25
amputations, 9, 12

anthocyanins, 58, 68
antioxidant, alphalipoic acid as, 106
apples, food tips on, 58
aspirin therapy, 15-16
    considerations, 16
atherosclerosis, 15, 58-59, 65

B

bagel recipes, 143-144, 205
Barrera, Joseph, MD, 17
beans, 58, 64, 79, 82, 83, 137-140
Benecol, 67
bioflavonoids, 66, 73
Blimpie menu items, 192
blindness, 9, 12
blood cholesterol, 50
blood glucose (sugar),

antioxidants and, 102
apples and soluble fiber and, 58
beans and, 83
control, 29-30, 47-49, 57
counting carbohydrates
    and, 84-85
foods and, 52-57
    breakfast, 56
    general eating plan, 55-56
    high fat vs. high
        carbohydrate, 55
    prevent higher blood
        sugars after meals,
        54-55
    when peak effects are
        shown, 53
foods that do not cause a
    rise in, 204
keeping a journal for, 84-86
lower fasting levels with
    alphalipoic acid, 106
monitoring, 7, 10, 13,
    44-45, 75, 110-111
peak after meal, 98
pizza and, 53-54, 84, 191
small meals and, 97-99
snacks and, 201-203
vitamin E and, 102-103
blood lipids, 49
    flaxseed and, 106
blood test (HgA1c), 49
    chromium and, 102
blood urea nitrogen (BUN), 39
body mass index (BMI), 27
Boston Market menu
    items, 189
bread, "white" vs. whole
    grain, 79

breakfast recipes, 140-145
Burger King, 72, 194
B-vitamins, food tips on, 58

C

caffeine in weight-loss
    products, 50
cake, nutrition information of
    mix vs. baked, 161
calcium, 58, 37
calories, avoiding in
    general, 183
cancer, 89, 106
cardiovascular disease, 9
Carl's Jr. menu items, 195
Centrum, 104-105
*Chez Moi—Lightening
    Up Recipes from Famous
    Restaurants*, 128
Chili's menu items, 186
chocolate, food tips on, 59
cholesterol, 51
    almonds and, 58
    dietary, 51
    food vs. blood, 50
    garlic and, 62
    HDL ("good"), 15, 40, 50, 58,
        63, 70, 73, 89
    heart disease and, 50
    isoflavones and, 63
    keeping low, 91-93
    LDL ("bad"), 15, 26, 49-51,
        58, 63, 65-67, 70-71,
        78, 80, 92
    lignans and, 64-65
    nuts and, 66

omega-3 fatty acid and, 89
plant stanol and sterol
    and, 67
psyllium and, 80
saturated fat and, 92
soluble fiber and, 71, 78
trans fats and, 70
walnuts and, 72
where to cut, 93
citrus, food tips on, 67
Complete Herbal, 107
coronary heart disease (CHD),
    nuts and, 66
Culpeper, Nicholas, 107
Cunnane, Stephen, Ph.D., 107

D

daily values, definition of, 159
dairy, food tips on, 59–60
Denny's menu items, 187-188
DHA (Docosahexaenoic
    acid), 60
diabetes,
    and heart disease, facts
        about, 57
    certified educator,
        finding, 16
    hotline, 16
    managing, 13
        three steps to, 7
diabetes *(see also type II
    diabetes),*
        gestational, 10
        type I, 11
diabetic neuropathy and
    alphalipoic acid, 106

dialysis, 39
diet,
    eating starchy foods and, 47
    fat in food and, 47-49
    high carbohydrate/very
        low-fat, 27
    high protein/low
        carbohydrate, 24-26,
46-47
    improving with
        supplements, 101-110
    moderate and balanced,
        27–28
    type II diabetes and, 43–52
dieting, 21-22
dietitian, finding a
    registered, 16
diets, high protein, 25-26
dyslipidemia, 14
dysmetabolic syndrome,
    see syndrome X.

E

eating plan, personalized,
    7, 14
eating,
    fight the urge at night, 100
    overindulging on holidays,
        121-122
    ways to lighten up the
        holidays, 122-124
edamame, food tips on, 60
eggs, food tips on, 60
    recipes using, 140-143
ephedra, 50
escarole, food tips on, 60

exercise
    and 4 reasons why many
        people don't, 112-115
    and variety, 113–114
    benefits, 29
    every little bit helps, 31
    getting started, 30
    home exercise equipment,
        32-33
    on holidays, 123
    recommendations, 111–112
    tips to keep you exercising,
        31-32

F

fast food, tips on, 68
fat, calculating grams of, 162
fat,
    as good or bad in food, 48-49
    avoiding when eating out,
        182-183
    cooking with, 90-91
    counting grams, 88-90
    definition of, 51
        hydrogenated, 51
        partially
          hydrogenated, 51
        monounsaturated, 51
        polyunsaturated, 52
        saturated, 52
    heart protective, 85, 87-91
    tips for limiting, 90
fat-related words, definitions
    of, 51-52
fatty acid, definition of, 51
Federal Trade Commission, 22
Flax Cookbook, The, 117

fiber,
    4 quick ways to get 30
        grams, 82-83
    appetite and, 81
    food tips on, 61
    function of in diet, 76-83
    side effects of, 81
fish, food tips on, 62
flavonoid, 59, 61, 63-64
flaxseed, 62, 68, 71, 82,
    106-110, 131-137
folic acid (folacin), 58, 60,
    61–62, 64, 67, 68
Food Steps to Freedom,
    the Ten, 75-115
food,
    journal, 84-86
    tips, 57-73
foods,
    menu selections at
        restaurants, 181-199
    well balanced and healthful
        supermarket selections,
        168-180
free, definition of, 158
fruit, 96-97
    nutrition tip, 211

G

garlic, food tips on, 62, 66
gas, 49
    fiber and, 81
genetics and diabetes, 10-12
gestational diabetes, 10
glycemic index,
    foods with a low, 206
    fruits with a low, 210

glycosylation, 102
*Good New Eating Plan for
    Type II Diabetes, The,* 12
guarana, 50

H

hazelnuts, food tips on, 62
HDL ("good") cholesterol,
    15, 40, 50, 58, 62–63, 70,
    73, 89
heart disease and diabetes,
    facts about, 57
HgA1c blood test, 49
    chromium and, 102
high blood pressure,
    see hypertension.
holidays, 121-124
homocysteine levels, 58,
    61–62
    and folic acid, 103
hummus recipe, 147
hydrogenated fat,
    definition of, 51
hydrogenated vegetable oils,
    food tips on, 63
hypertension, 34-37, 41, 59,
    65, 102

I

insulin, 10-11, 29, 77, 101
    whole-grain snacks and, 202
iron, 104
isoflavones, 63, 64

J

Jack in the Box menu
    items, 195
JELL-O, 179
jicama, food tips on, 63–64

K

kale, food tips on, 64
Kentucky Fried Chicken
    menu items, 196
kidney beans, food tips on, 64
kidney failure, 9

L

lactobacillus acidophilus, 73
LDL ("bad") cholesterol, 15,
    26, 49-51, 58, 63, 65-67,
    70-71, 78, 80, 92
light, definition of, 158
Lighten Up!, 117, 129
lignans, 64, 107
lipids, blood, 49
lipolysis, 10
lipoprotein (a), 65
lipoproteins, 70
    definition of, 52
Lp(a), *see lipoprotein (a).*
lycopene, 64, 69

M

magnesium, 37, 65, 102
    nuts and, 66

margarine, food tips on, 65

McDonald's, 65, 196

meals,
> small,
>> benefits of, 97-99
>> frequency of, 99
>> snacks and, 201-202
>> medication and insulin
>> and, 101

meat loaf recipe, 154

medication and meals, 101

metabolic syndrome, 65

monounsaturated fat,
> canola oil and, 59, 87
> definition of, 51
> hazelnuts and, 63
> olive oil and, 66, 88
> walnuts and, 72

N

National Center for Health
> Statistics, 20

National Eye Institute, 12

nectarines, food tips on, 66

neuropoathy
> and alphalipoic acid, 106

nutrient, 105

nutrition information,
> misleading, 161

nuts,
> food tips on, 66
> nutrition tip, 207

O

oatmeal recipes, 144, 149

Olive Garden menu items, 190

olive oil,
> fats and, 88, 90-91
> food tips on, 65

omega-3 fatty acids,
> food tips on, 66
> information about, 89
> plant omega-3s, 67

omega-3 recipes, 150-153

onions, food tips on, 66

orange juice, food tips on,
> 64, 67

oranges, food tips on, 67

overeating, 121-124, 160

P

partially hydrogenated fat,
> definition of, 51

personalized eating plan, 7, 14

phenolics, 58

phytoestrogen, 58, 64, 107

phytosterols, 58, 66

pizza, 53-54, 84, 191

plant omega-3s, 67, 72

plant stanol, food tips on, 67

plant sterol, food tips on, 67

platelet abnormality, 15

polyphenols, 67, 71

polyunsaturated fat, 52

potassium, 37

potato recipes, 124-126, 139

produce, food tips on, 67

psyllium, 67–68, 80, 83

pumpkin pie recipe, 129–130

Q

quercetin, 68
quick entrée recipes, 153-155

R

raspberries, food tips on, 68
Recipe Doctor, The, 117
recipes,
    26 you can't live without,
      117-156
      3-minute burrito, 138
      apple lover's oatmeal,
        144–145
      best cornbread
        dressing, 128
      easy 3-bean salad, 146
      easy omega-3 fatty acid
        tuna sandwich, 152–153
      egg muffin sandwich
        lite, 141–143
      flaxseed focaccia, 133
      flaxseed jam
        muffins, 132
      flaxseed maple scones, 135
      green bean casserole, 126
      hash brown casserole, 125
      high legume fried
        rice, 137
      honey wheat bread with
        flaxseed, 131
      iced café mocha, 148
      lemon dijon salmon,
        150–151
      light and flaky
        buttermilk pie
        crust, 130
      light club sandwich, 155

      light Denver omelette
        for two, 140
      light Libby's
        pumpkin pie, 129
      lox-ness monster bagel
        spread, 143–144
      monounsaturated
        side salad, 145
      oat bran meat loaf,
        153–154
      oatmeal raisin bites,
        149–150
      pintos and cheese, 139
      potato latkes, 124
      quick-fix chili and
        fries, 139
      quick ranch dip (with
        vegetables), 146–147
      simple salmon
        pasta salad, 151–152
      spicy hummus with
        crudites and
        crackers, 147–148
      sun-dried tomato pesto
        bagel spread, 143
    substitutions in 117-121,
      123-124
reduced, definition of, 158
renal disease, 12
restaurant rules to eat by,
    181-199
    cutting fat and calories
      when eating out, 182-183
    good choices at pizza
      parlors, 190-191
    good choices at sandwich
      shops, 192
    good choices at fast food
      chains, 192-197

menu items,
bagel shops, 198
Blimpie, 192
Boston Market, 189
Burger King, 194
Carl's Jr., 195
Chili's, 186
Denny's, 187-188
donut/coffee shop chain,
198–199
Jack in the Box, 195
Kentucky Fried
Chicken, 196
McDonald's, 196
Olive Garden, 190
steakhouse chain,
184-185
Subway, 192-193
Wendy's, 197
restaurants, food tips on, 68
risk factors for type II
diabetes, 10

S

salmon recipes, 151-152
salt, 38
saponins, 58
saturated fat,
definition of, 52
food tips on, 68
sources of, 92
trying to keep low, 91-93
selenium, 103
food tips on, 68–69
serving sizes, 157-158
side dish recipes, 145-146
Slim Fast, 20

snack and pick-me-up recipes,
146-150
snacks,
smart recipes,
bagel and cream
cheese, 205
"Healthy Pop" Jolly Time
popcorn, 211
melon medley, 209
mini turkey melts,
209-210
peanut butter banana
fana, 205-206
pear and jarlsburg
lite, 209
quick vegetable bean
salad, 206-207
strawberry lemonade
smoothie, 203
Wendy's side salad, 21
yogurt parfait, 208
smart selection, 201-211
when appropriate at
bedtime, 100
sodium, sensitivity to, 38
soluble fiber, 45-46,
76-83
benefits of, 76-77
flaxseed and, 108
food tips on, 71
how it works, 77-78
psyllium and, 68
snacks with, 202
tips for incorporating into
meals, 78
where to find, 79-80
soy, food tips on, 69
stanol, food tips on, 67
starchy foods, 47

sterol, food tips on, 67

strawberries, food tips on, 69

substitutions in recipes, 117-121, 123-124

Subway menu items, 192-193

sugars, other names for, 159

supplements,
flaxseed, 106-110
multivitamins and
minerals as,
antioxidants, 102
chromium, 102
folic acid, 103
iron, 104
magnesium, 102
questions to ask about, 103-104
selenium, 103
vitamin C, 102
vitamin E, 102, 104-106

syndrome X, 40-41, 72
criteria T, 40-41

Take Control, 67

tea, food tips on, 69

Tell Me What to Eat series, 5-6

T

thiosulfinates, 67

thromboxane synthesis, 15

tocopherol, 66, 105

tofu, food tips on, 69

tomatoes, food tips on, 69

trans fats,
coronary heart disease
and, 70

food tips on, 69–70

trans fatty acids, definition
of, 52

triglycerides, 16, 29, 40, 49, 62, 77

tuna sandwich recipe, 152–153

type I diabetes, 11

type II diabetes,
ethnicity and, 10
genetic predisposition, 11-12
Top 7 profiles
A diabetic on dialysis, 39
Hyper about
hypertension, 34-37
I have couch potato-itis, 29-34
Salt movers and
shakers, 38
Syndrome X–Y me, 40-41
Type II and thin, 38-39
Waiting to lose weight, 20-29
warning signs of, 11

U

umbelliferous vegetables, food
tips on, 70

unsaturated fats,
food tips on, 70
nuts and, 66

V

vascular thrombosis, 15

vegetable oils, food tips on, 70

vegetables, making more convenient, 96-97
vegetarian entrées, food tips on, 71
vegetarianism, 45
viscous fiber, *see soluble fiber.*
vitamin C,
    food tips on, 71
    glycosylation and, 102
vitamin E, supplementing, 104-105
    warning, 104–105

fact, 23
products using dangerous substances, 50
what to look for in a diet, 28
Weight Watchers, 20
weight, national U.S. increase, 20
Wendy's menu items, 197
wholegrains, food tips on, 71–72
whole-wheat tortillas, food tips on, 72

walnuts, food tips on, 71
weight loss,
    benefits, 14
    body fat vs. lean body mass or body water, 24
    facilitating, 21-22

yogurt, food tips on, 73
    nutrition tip, 208

Z

zucchini, food tips on, 73

About the Author

E laine Magee, M.P.H., R.D., is an anti-dieting dietitian who believes we should all eat and exercise for "the health of it" and let the pounds fall where they may. Elaine describes herself as "fit, fabulous, and fourteen" (size 14, that is).

Elaine graduated as the Nutrition and Food Science Department's Student of the Year from San José State University with a B.S. in nutrition and a minor in chemistry. She also obtained her master's degree in public health nutrition from UC Berkeley and is a registered dietitian. She was a nutrition instructor at Diablo Valley College for two years and the nutrition marketing specialist (California Department of Health) for the now national "5 a Day" health program for three years. Several of the brochures she developed for the program won awards in health education.

Elaine's credits include:

- Best-selling author. Elaine has written more than 26 books since her first book was released in 1989.

- Newspaper columnist. Called the "Dear Abby of cooking," Elaine writes "The Recipe Doctor," which is now available to newspapers across the country through Knight Ridder/Tribune Information Services. In her column, Elaine "doctors" real recipes to make them more nutritious, while retaining the original good taste.

- WebMD nutrition expert. Elaine currently writes articles for WebMD, is the guest author on at least one "chat" a month, and is the nutrition expert for two WebMD message/information boards: "Healthy Cooking—Special Needs" and WebMD Weight Loss Clinic's "Recipe Doctor Board."

- Magazine journalist. Elaine is a regular contributor to *Woman's Day* and *All You* magazines. She has also written articles and recipe features for *Cooking Light, Dance Spirit, American Girl*, and *Parenting*.

- TV personality. Elaine recently conducted monthly "Recipe Doctor" nutrition/cooking segments on the Greater San Francisco Bay Area NBC affiliate's Saturday morning news show. For two years, Elaine performed the "Light Cooking" segment for the KSBW-TV (NBC) midday news in Salinas, California. She has appeared on *CBS Evening News*, CNN, *Caryl & Marilyn: Real Friends, Good Morning New York*, and *The Debra Duncan Show*, as well as local television shows in the Pacific Northwest.

- Public speaker. Elaine has lectured at multiple local and national conferences. She has most recently appeared as a speaker at the "Kid's Artistic Review Dance" convention in New York

City, "Speaking of Women's Health" conference in San José, the "Matters of the Heart" American Heart Association conference in California, and the "To Your Health for a Change" Woman Kind conference in San Francisco.

Elaine has her own Web site (www.recipedoctor.com), making it easy for readers of her national column to submit recipe-doctoring requests, find out more about her books, and learn about her passion for cooking with children.